NURSING

The Philosophy and Science of Caring

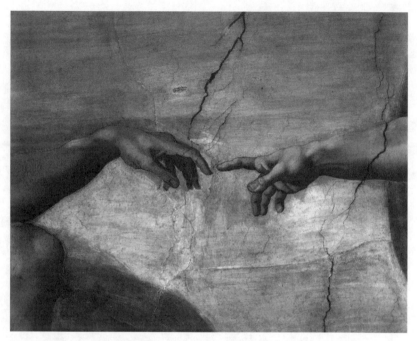

Figure 1: Frontispiece: The Creation of Adam: *detail of the hands of God and Adam, by Michelangelo Buonarroti (1475–1564). Detail of the ceiling of the Sistine Chapel, Vatican Palace, State of the Vatican City. Photo credit: Scala / Art Resource, New York.*

NURSING
The Philosophy and Science of Caring
REVISED EDITION

JEAN WATSON, PHD, RN, AHC-BC, FAAN

Distinguished Professor of Nursing
Murchinson-Scoville Endowed Chair in Caring Science
University of Colorado–Denver, Anschutz Medical Center
Aurora

UNIVERSITY PRESS OF COLORADO

Published by the University Press of Colorado
5589 Arapahoe Avenue, Suite 206C
Boulder, Colorado 80303

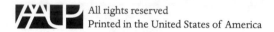

The University Press of Colorado is a proud member of
the Association of American University Presses.

The University Press of Colorado is a cooperative publishing enterprise supported, in part,
by Adams State College, Colorado State University, Fort Lewis College, Mesa State College,
Metropolitan State College of Denver, University of Colorado, University of Northern
Colorado, and Western State College of Colorado.

∞ The paper used in this publication meets the minimum requirements of the American
National Standard for Information Sciences—Permanence of Paper for Printed Library
Materials. ANSI Z39.48-1992

Library of Congress Cataloging-in-Publication Data

Watson, Jean, 1940–
    Nursing : the philosophy and science of caring / Jean Watson. — Rev. ed.
        p. ; cm.
    Includes bibliographical references and index.
    ISBN 978-0-87081-898-1 (pbk. : alk. paper) 1. Nursing—Philosophy. 2. Nursing—Psy-
chological aspects. 3. Nurse and patient. 4. Helping behavior. I. Title.
    [DNLM: 1. Nurse-Patient Relations. 2. Nursing Care—methods. 3. Philosophy, Nurs-
ing. WY 87 W3393n 2008]
    RT84.5.W37 2008
    610.7301—dc22
                                                                    2008001410

17   16   15   14   13   12   11   10   09   10   9   8   7   6   5   4

This new edition is dedicated to my grandchildren, Demitri, Alma, and Theo Ervedosa and Gabriel and Joseph Willis. My gratitude and love to my beautiful daughters, Jennifer and Julie. I am so blessed to have them in my life and my life's work; they are often my best teachers. I also wish to honor the teachings, support, and lessons learned from my late husband, Douglas, who was with me for the duration of the writing of the first edition of this book.

The students at the University of Colorado, and students and colleagues around the world, continue to inspire and inform me about the deeper nature of this work and its potential for generating love and caring globally, opening new horizons for caring, healing, and peace in the world. I am always learning from these inspirited others who make this framework a living presence in their personal and professional lives in nursing and health care.

The focus of this work is not for every nurse but for the Caritas Nurse *who is on the journey toward the deeper caring-healing dimensions of nursing and is on the personal-professional path of authenticity and evolution of consciousness, bringing Love, Spirit, purpose, and meaning back into his/her life and life's work in the world.*

This work serves somewhat as a continuing message to the next generation of nurses and health practitioners engaged in and committed to Caritas *practices. My special gratitude goes to those students, practitioners, and colleagues around the world who are being and doing "The Work." As I often say, I sit at your feet in awe.*

I also remind all: I write and teach what I am learning, needing continually to learn.

Kathryn Lynch, an advanced nursing student and my research associate at the University of Colorado–Denver and Rush Presbyterian University, is specially acknowledged as a gift to me during the writing of this book. She has offered her talents to support me and my activities and requests related to this book and also to other professional work emerging from my writings. She has created new templates for my Web site (www.uchsc.edu/nursing/caring) and helped to update and maintain it.

Further, she has served as Web master and assistant to the emerging international group, the International Caritas Consortium (www.caritasconsortium.org), whose members convene to share their work in this area, learn from each other, and offer guidance to others who wish to pursue this Caring Science/*Caritas* model as a direction for their professional and personal lives and work.

I want to recognize and thank Darrin Pratt and the University Press of Colorado for their continuing interest and support in keeping this work alive and updated for a new generation of faculty, students, and practitioners. This new, revised edition seeks to keep the caring-healing values, concepts, hopes, and vision alive in the world for all those committed to a Philosophy and Science of Human Caring as the foundation for nursing and health care and for sustaining humanity itself.

Opening-Entering: A New Beginning Almost Thirty Years Later

I sit in the quiet of Mexico, my secret, sacred space, on my birthday with a sense of nostalgia and my questionable notions of life and cycles of time. I sit in the quiet, reengaging with my very first book on the philosophy and science of caring in nursing. The original work (1979) presented this framework as the foundation, the soul, the core and essence of nursing as a discipline and a profession.

I now ponder a total renewal, revision, and update of this work, bringing life to it at this point in time, having undergone and experienced several life evolutions, changes, even transformations of self and systems, including the deepening of the "theory."

I reconnect with my life cycle as well as the career cycles of my work, both as the beginning and ending and as the continuing cycle of this time. Just as the high tide comes at noon and the low tide recedes at sunset, I place myself with the rhythm of the sea. My mood is in harmony with the ocean swells as they rise and fall with each cycle of the waves. So, I prepare to revise and update this original work as I come full circle in reviewing my life, my work, and my career, moving to another rhythmic space for this time in my personal and professional life world.

Or rather, I let it all move me, take me, wash over me, prepare me for a new space in my thinking and reconnecting—like a new wave upon the shore, yet with familiarity of the oceanic sea-of-thinking, which still runs through my life and my collected work on caring. I am continually writing, teaching, pondering what I need to learn.

Not knowing how this revised edition will unfold but open to its emergence, I invite others to enter into and follow my path into the future. At this moment I am both somber and celebratory as I journey into the process.

Caring begins with being present, open to compassion, mercy, gentleness, loving-kindness, and equanimity toward and with self before one can offer compassionate caring to others. It begins with a love of humanity and everything that is living: the immanent, subtle, radiant, shadow-and-light vicissitudes of experiences along the way— honoring with reverence the mystery, the unknowns, the impermanence and changes but actively, joyfully participating in all of it, the pain, the joy, and everything.

Thus, to begin, I invite you to enter into a centering, mindful process, a reflective pause, and a contemplative meditation:

> Just take a deep breath and appreciate yourself, your life, in all its fullness/emptiness, whatever you are feeling just now, pondering briefly what is emerging for you in relation to your personal calling into nursing and your continuing reason and purpose for remaining. I invite you to briefly dwell in silence, open your heart as well as your mind; offer a sense of gratitude for your life and all that has brought you to this point in time.

Thus, you begin to realize with this entering space of pause, silence, breath, and gratitude that this evolved work is more than a new edition of an original work; it evokes a contemplative, reflective quieting down. This work invites a return to one's inner core to

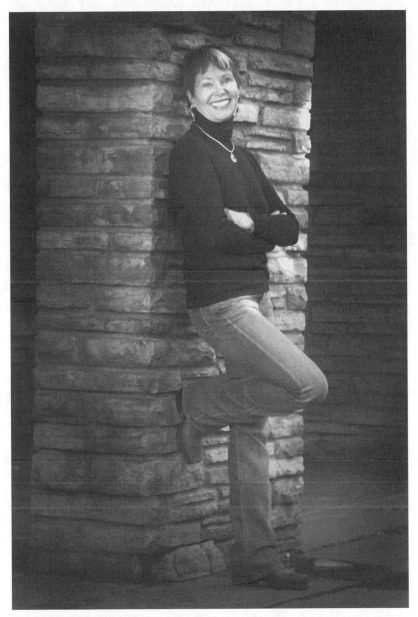

Figure 2. Jean Watson (author) in Boulder, Colorado, on University of Colorado campus. Photo by AliveStudios.com.

reconnect with the timeless collective foundation and very soul of this ancient, pioneering, and noble profession.

It is hoped that this continuing work will arouse a remembering of why you entered this field, reconnecting with what is keeping you involved and the knowledge, values, and practices that are essential if you, other nurses, and nursing itself are to sustain the enduring and timeless gift of offering informed, moral, knowledgeable, compassionate human caring-healing services to sustain humanity in our daily work and in the world.

I am truly honored and blessed because you are part of my journey. I thank you for being a sojourner on this path.

JW

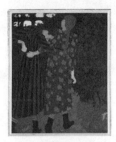

Figure 3. Young Girls Walking *by Edouard Vuillard, c. 1891.*

INTERLUDE

You/We who do not know the future of nursing and health care
We/You who know too much of the past
Now step into new space
You/We create new options
Envision new hopes
And possibilities not yet dreamt of—
Vibrating possibilities
Waiting to unfold for humanity, for health, for healing
For Being-Doing-Becoming Nursing in a new tune.
Learning a new song—
A new sound, a new rhythm, a new Voice
Opening to that which might be, not conforming to what already is
And which no longer serves
Self, society
You/We the old and new
As you encounter anyone who tells you
Nursing is less than what you know and believe
Bless them and turn away.
If what anyone tells you is fear-based, limited, or limiting
Also bless them and turn away.
Turn toward love and caring from own deep self.
You are the source of your own power and possibilities

JW

PART I

Background

Nursing: The Philosophy and Science of Caring (1979) was my first book and my entrance into scholarly work. This book was published before formal attention was being given to nursing theory as the foundation for the discipline of nursing and before much focus had been directed to a meaningful philosophical foundation for nursing science, education, and practice.

The work "emerged from my quest to bring new meaning and dignity to the work and the world of nursing and patient care" (Watson 1997:49). The theoretical concepts were derived and emerged from my personal and professional experiences; they were clinically inducted, empirically grounded, and combined with my philosophical, ethical, intellectual, and experiential background (Watson 1997). My quest and my work have always been about deepening my own and everyone's understanding of humanity and life itself and bringing those dimensions into nursing. Thus, the early work emerged from my own values, beliefs, perceptions, and experience with rhetorical and ineffable questions. For example, what does it mean to be human? What does it mean to care? What does it mean to heal? Questions and views of personhood, life, the birth-death cycle, change, health, healing, relationships, caring, wholeness, pain, suffering, humanity itself, and other unknowns guided my quest to identify a framework for nursing as a distinct entity, profession, discipline, and science in its own right—separate from, but complementary to, the curative orientation of medicine (Watson 1979). My views were heightened by my commitment to (1) the professional role and mission of nursing; (2) its ethical covenant with society as sustaining human caring and preserving human dignity, even when threatened; and (3) attending to and helping to sustain human dignity, humanity, and wholeness in the midst of threats and crises of life and death. All these activities, experiences, questions, and processes transcend illness, diagnosis, condition, setting, and so on; they were, and remain, enduring and timeless across time and space and changes in systems, society, civilization, and science.

The original (1979) work has expanded and evolved through a generation of publications, other books, videos, and CDs, along with clinical-educational and administrative initiatives for transforming professional nursing. A series of other books on caring theory followed and have been translated into at least nine languages. The other major theory-based books on caring that followed the original work include:

- *Nursing: Human Science and Human Care. A Theory of Nursing* (1985). East Norwick, CT: Appleton-Century-Crofts. Reprinted/ republished (1988). New York: National League for Nursing. Reprinted/republished (1999). Sudbury, MA: Jones & Bartlett.

- *Postmodern Nursing and Beyond* (1999). Edinburgh, Scotland: Churchill-Livingstone. Reprinted/republished New York: Elsevier.

- *Assessing and Measuring Caring in Nursing and Health Science* (ed.) (2002). New York: Springer (AJN Book of Year award).

- *Caring Science as Sacred Science* (2005). Philadelphia: F. A. Davis (AJN Book of Year award).

Other caring-based books I coedited or coauthored are extensions of these works but are not discussed here (see, for example, Bevis and Watson [1989], *Toward a Caring Curriculum*, New York: National League for Nursing [reprinted 1999, Sudbury, MA: Jones & Bartlett]; Watson and Ray [1998] [eds.], *The Ethics of Care and the Ethics of Care*, New York: National League for Nursing; Chinn and Watson [1994], *Art and Aesthetics in Nursing*, New York: National League for Nursing). See also Web site (Watson 2004a) for complete citations of books and publications.

Nursing: The Philosophy and Science of Caring (1979) provided the original core and structure for the Theory of Human Caring: Ten Carative Factors. These factors were identified as the essential aspects of caring in nursing, without which nurses may not have been practicing professional nursing but instead were functioning as technicians or skilled workers within the dominant framework of medical techno-cure science. This work has stood as a timeless classic of sorts on its own. It has not been revised since its original publication; only reprints have kept it alive, thanks to the University Press of Colorado.

This (2008) edition is an expanded and updated supplement of the original text, with completely new sections replacing previous sections while other sections that remain relevant are included with only minor revisions. I have been advised to retain the original text in this revision so essential parts of it remain alive, since the original 1979 version may eventually go out of print. Thus, this work retains core essentials of the original text while updating that text with new content, bringing the original book full circle with my own evolution and changes in the work across an almost thirty-year span.

To provide the context for this evolution (before I address revisions of the original text), I provide a brief overview of the focus and content of the other books that serve as a background for my evolving work, all of which emerged from the original text of *Nursing: The Philosophy and Science of Caring*.

My second book, *Nursing: Human Science and Human Care, A Theory of Nursing*, was first published in 1985 and has been republished by the National League for Nursing (1988) and Jones and Bartlett (1999). It expands on the philosophical, transpersonal aspects of a caring moment as the core framework. This focus places the theoretical ideas more explicitly within a broader context of ethics, art, and even metaphysics as phenomena within which nursing dwells but often does not name, articulate, or act upon.

As has been pointed out in contemporary postmodern thinking, if a profession does not have its own language, it does not exist; thus, it is important to name, claim, articulate, and act upon the phenomena of nursing and caring if nursing is to fulfill its mandate and raison d'être for society. This second theory text seeks to make more explicit the reality that if nursing is to survive in this millennium, it has to sustain and make explicit its covenant with the public. This covenant includes taking mature professional responsibility for giving voice to, standing up for, and acting on its knowledge, values, ethics, and skilled practices of caring, healing, and health.

What was/is prominent in the second "theory" book is the explicit acknowledgment of the spiritual dimensions of caring and healing. There is further development of concepts such as the transpersonal, the caring occasion, the caring moment, and the "art of transpersonal caring" (Watson 1985:67). Further, in this work, as reflected in the title, distinctions are made with respect to the context of human science in which nursing resides: for example,

- A philosophy of human freedom, choice, responsibility
- A biology and psychology of holism
- An epistemology that allows not only for empirics but also for the advancement of aesthetics, ethical values, intuition, personal knowing, spiritual insights, along with a process of discovery, creative imagination, evolving forms of inquiry
- An ontology of time *and* space
- A context of inter-human events, processes, and relationships that connect/are one with the environment and the wider universe
- A scientific worldview that is open. (Watson 1985:16)

Thus, a human science and human caring orientation differs from conventional science and invites qualitatively different aspects to be honored as legitimate and necessary when working with human experiences and human caring-healing, health, and life phenomena.

In this work one finds the first mention of "caring occasion," "pheno-menal field," "transpersonal," and the "art of transpersonal caring," inviting the full use of self within a "caring moment" (Watson 1985: 58–72). The caring occasion / caring moment becomes transpersonal when "two persons (nurse and other) together with their unique life histories and phenomenal field (of perception) become a focal point in space and time, from which the moment has a field of its own that is greater than the occasion itself. As such, the process can (and does) go beyond itself, yet arise from aspects of itself that become part of the life history of each person, as well as part of some larger, deeper, com-plex pattern of life" (Watson 1985:59).

The caring moment can be an existential turning point for the nurse, in that it involves pausing, choosing to "see"; it is informed action guided by an intentionality and consciousness of how to *be* in the moment—fully present, open to the other person, open to compas-sion and connection, beyond the ego-control focus that is so common. In a caring moment, the nurse grasps the gestalt of the presenting moment and is able to "read" the field, beyond the outer appearance of the patient and the patient's behavior. The moment is "transper-sonal" when the nurse is able to see and connect with the spirit of oth-ers, open to expanding possibilities of what can occur. The foundation for this perspective is the wisdom in knowing and understanding that "[w]e learn from one another how to be more human by identifying ourselves with others and finding their dilemmas in ourselves. What we all learn from it is self-knowledge. The self we learn about or dis-cover is every self: it is universal. We learn to recognize ourselves in others" (Watson 1985:59).

This human-to-human connection expands our compassion and caring and keeps alive our common humanity. All of this process deepens and sustains our shared humanity and helps to avoid reducing another human being to the moral status of object (Watson 1985:60).

This second work concludes with a sample of human science meth-odology as a form of caring inquiry. Transcendental phenomenology is discussed as one exemplar of a human science–Caring Science experi-ence of loss and grief experienced and researched among an Aboriginal tribe in Western Australia. Poetry and artistic, metaphoric expressions

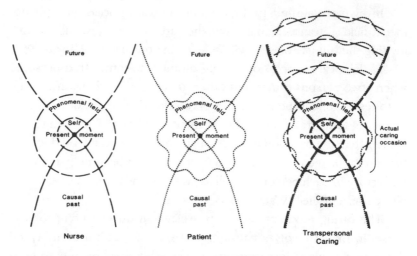

Figure 4. Dynamics of Human Caring Process, Including Nurse-Patient Transpersonal Dimension. Illustration by Mel Gabel, University of Colorado, Biomedical Communications Department. Reprinted, with permission, from Watson (1985/1999).

emerge within the "outback" research experience, using this extended methodology. Such an approach was consistent with the findings and experiences in this unique setting, in that this methodology allowed for a "poetic" effect in articulating experiences as felt and lived, transcending their facts and pure descriptions (descriptive phenomenology).

Thus, the transcendent views were consistent with transpersonal dimensions and provided space for paradox, ambiguity, sensuous resonance, and creative expressions, going beyond the surface phenomenology (Watson 1985:90–91). For example: "In other words, how could cold, unfeeling, totally detached dogmatic words and tone possibly teach the truth or deep meaning of a human phenomenon associated with human caring, transpersonal caring and grief, and convey experiences of great sorrow, great beauty, passion and joy. We cannot convey the need for compassion, complexity, or for cultivating feeling and sensibility in words that are bereft of warmth, kindness and good feeling" (Watson 1985:91). The result is poetizing; "it cannot be other than poetic" (Heidegger quoted in Watson 1985:98).

Such an exemplar of methodology invites a union between the humanities and art with science, one of the perennial themes of my work. Finally, this second book launched my ideas and set the foundation for the next evolution of my work on Caring Science that followed.

The third book, *Postmodern Nursing and Beyond* (1999), brought focus to the professional paradigm that is grounded in the ontology of relations and an ethical-ontological foundation before jumping to the epistemology of science and technology. The focus of this work was the need to clarify the ontological foundation of Being-in-Relation within a caring paradigm, the unity of mind-body-spirit/field, going beyond the outdated separatist ontology of modern Era I medical-industrial thinking. In this book the spiritual and evolved energetic aspects of caring consciousness, intentionality, and human presence and the personal evolution of the practitioner became more developed. This evolution was placed within the emerging postmodern cosmology of healing, wholeness, and oneness that is an honoring of the unity of all.

This postmodern perspective, as developed in the third book, attempts to project nursing and health care into the mid-twenty-first century, when there will be radically different requirements for all health practitioners and entirely different roles and expectations between and among the public and health care systems (Watson 1999: xiii). Prominent in this text is an emphasis on the feminine yin energy needed for caring and healing, which nursing, other practitioners, and society alike are rediscovering because the dominant system is imbalanced with the archetypal energy of yang, which is not the source for healing. Nursing itself serves as an archetype for healing and represents a metaphor for the deep yin healing energy that is emerging within an entirely different paradigm. What is proposed is a fundamental ontological shift in consciousness, acknowledging a symbiotic relationship between humankind-technology-nature and the larger, expanding universe. This evolutionary turn evokes a return to the sacred core of humankind, inviting mystery and wonder back into our lives, work, and world. Such views reintroduce a sense of reverence for and openness to infinite possibilities. Emphasis is placed on the importance of ontological caring-healing practices, grounded in an expanded consciousness and intentionality that intersect with techno-logical treatments of advanced medicine. In this work, Nightingale's original blueprint for nursing is evident and embodies all the caring-healing nursing arts and rituals, rediscovered and honored for new reasons. Metaphors of *ontological archetype, ontological artist, and ontological architect* are used to capture the roles and visions for nursing into this millennium/Era III medicine and nursing (Watson 1999:xiv–xv).

My most recent theoretical book, *Caring Science as Sacred Science* (2005) (which received an *American Journal of Nursing* [AJN] Book of the Year award in 2006 in the category of research), expands further upon the earlier works on caring. This work places Caring Science within an ethical–moral–philosophically evolved, scientific context, guided by the works of Emmanual Levinas (1969, French) and Knud Logstrup (1997, Danish).

This latest work on Caring Science seeks a science model that reintegrates metaphysics within the material physical domain and reinvites Ethics-of-Belonging (to the infinite field of Universal Cosmic Love) (Levinas 1969) as before and underneath *Being-by-Itself* alone—no longer separate from the broader universal field of infinity to which we all belong and to which we return from the earth plane.

Levinas's "Ethics of face"—as in facing our own and others' humanity—is explored as a metaphor for how we deepen and sustain our humanity for survival of the human, in contrast to "totalizing" the human condition and cutting us off from the infinite source of life and the great Cosmic field that unites us all. Logstrup's "ethical demand" brings forth the notion of "Ethics of Hand," in that he reminds us of the sovereign, unarticulated, and often anonymous ethical demand that "we take care of the life which trust has placed in our hands" (Logstrup 1997:18).

Caring Science as Sacred Science text identifies these basic assumptions (Watson 2005:56):

- The Infinity of the Human Spirit and evolving universe
- The ancient and emerging cosmology of a unity consciousness of relatedness of All

- The ontological ethic of *Belonging before Our Separate Being* (Levinas 1969)

- The moral position of sustaining the infinity and mystery of the human condition and keeping alive the evolving human spirit across time, as in *facing and deepening our own and others' Humanity* (Levinas 1969)

- The ethical demand that acknowledges that we hold another person's life in our hands; this sovereign expression of life is given to us, before and beyond our control with expressions of trust, love, caring, honesty, forgiveness, gratitude, and so on, beyond ego fixations and obsessive feelings that are negative expressions of life (Logstrup 1997)

- The relationship between our consciousness, words, and thoughts and how they positively or negatively affect our energetic-transpersonal field of Being, Becoming, and Belonging; thus, our consciousness affects our ability to connect, to "be-in-right-relation" with Source: the infinite universal Cosmic field of LOVE.

In this evolved context of Caring Science, we can appreciate, honor, and face the reality that life is given to us as a gift; we are invited to sustain and deepen our own and others' humanity as our moral and ethical starting point for professional caring-healing. In Levinas's view, "Ethics of Belonging" (to this universal field of Cosmic Love) becomes the first principle and starting point for any science, allowing ethics and metaphysics to be reunited with conventional science.

These views are not unlike Nightingale's notion of natural healing processes, which draw upon spiritual dimensions that are the greatest source of healing (1969). Indeed, it has been acknowledged in perennial philosophies and Wisdom Traditions across time, cultures, and a diversity of belief systems that the greatest source of healing is love.

Thus, my book on Caring Science brings a decidedly sacred dimension to the work of caring, making more explicit that we dwell in mystery and the infinity of Cosmic Love as the source and depth of all of life.

We come from the spirit world and return to the spirit source when vulnerable, stressed, fearful, ill, and so forth. This is comparable to

Nightingale's notion of putting the patient in best condition for nature to heal, acknowledging that healing draws on nature and natural processes. In this framework it is acknowledged that we are working with the inner life forces, life energy, and the soul, if you will, of self and other and that we need to connect with the universal infinite field.

> A human being is a part of the whole called the "universe," a part limited in time and space. He [sic] experiences [self], thoughts and feelings, as something separated from the rest, a kind of optical illusion . . . of consciousness. . . . Our task must be to free ourselves from this prison [of illusion] by widening our circle of compassion [love and caring] to embrace all living creatures and the whole of nature in all its beauty. Nobody is able to achieve this completely, but the striving for such achievement is in itself part of the liberation. (Albert Einstein quoted on title page of Williamson 2002)

When we are conscious of an expanded cosmology and an expanded, deeper moral-ethical foundation, we gain new insights and awakenings; we open to the sense of humanity-in-relation-to-the-larger-universe, inspiring a sense of wonder, wisdom, awe, and humility. We are invited to accept our need for wisdom, beyond information and knowledge alone, and to surrender to both that which is greater than our separate ego-self and the outer world we think we have control over and seek to manipulate.

In the present work I reassert the emerging, evolving wonder at and appreciation for viewing the human-universe as One. The holographic view of caring mirrors the holographic universe: that is, the whole is in each part, and each part affects the whole.

So, in developing concepts and practices, theories and philosophies of caring-healing that intersect with Love, we invoke Caring as part of our consciousness and intention to affect the whole with practical engagement from our own unique gifts and talents. In doing so, our part of personal and professional work is contributing to and making a difference in the moment but is also affecting the holographic universal field that surrounds us and to which we all belong.

In other words, through modern science as well as through ancient wisdom traditions, we realize that what we do for ourselves benefits others and what we do for others benefits us. If one person is healed, it is helping to heal all. If others are healed, it helps us heal. The mutuality of Caring affects the universal field to which we all belong, and we energetically affect it with our consciousness and our concrete acts. We all are candidates for awakening a compassionate heart (Chödrön 2005), the deeper foundation for *Caritas Nursing*.

I now, thirty years later, after offering an overview and update of the previous texts of my evolved work in Caring Science and the Theory of Human Caring, turn back to the original text and offer revisions and current perspectives for the new edition. Ironically, and perhaps not surprisingly, the original text held the blueprint for the evolution of these ideas that have both sustained and expanded over these years.

PART II

Caring Science as Context

CHAPTER ONE

NURSING: THE PHILOSOPHY AND SCIENCE OF CARING

Revised Edition

The original text begins with a discussion of nursing as the Philosophy and Science of Caring. I now ponder suggesting that today, almost thirty years later, it perhaps could equally be framed as *Caring: The Philosophy and Science of Nursing*. Discussions and ambiguity remain as to the nature of Caring Science and its relation to nursing science. Rhetorical questions arise, such as, are there distinct differences between the two? Do they overlap? Do they intersect? Are they one and the same? These questions perhaps remain, but the present work offers a distinct position. By transposing the order of Nursing and Caring, it invites a new discourse and context.

My position is this: Caring Science as a starting point for nursing as a field of study offers a distinct disciplinary foundation for the profession; it provides an ethical, moral, values-guided meta-narrative for its science and its human phenomena, its approach to caring-healing-person-nature-universe. It reintroduces spirit and sacred dimensions back into our work and life and world. It allows for a reunion between metaphysics and the material-physical world of modern science.

In positing Caring Science as the disciplinary context and matrix that guides professional development and maturity, I acknowledge that there is a difference between the discipline of nursing and the profession of nursing. It is widely known that the discipline (of any field) should inform the profession. The disciplinary matrix of Caring carries the meta-paradigm, the values, the metaphysics, the philosophical-moral meta-narrative with respect to what it means to be human, honoring unity of Being, the oneness of mind-body-spirit/universe; the discipline offers subject matter foci and a distinct perspective on the subject matter. The profession, without clarity of its disciplinary context, loses its way in the midst of the outer-worldly changes and forces for conformity to the status quo of the moment.

The discipline of nursing, from my position, is/should be grounded in Caring Science; this, in turn, informs the profession. Caring Science informs and serves as the moral-philosophical-theoretical-foundational starting point for nursing education, patient care, research, and even administrative practices.

If nursing across time had been born and matured within the consciousness and clarity of a Caring Science orientation, perhaps it would be in a very different evolved place today: a place beyond the struggles with conventional biomedical-technical science that linger still, beyond the crisis in care that haunts hospitals and systems today, beyond the critical shortage of nurses and nursing that society is experiencing at this turn in history, and beyond the noncaring communities in our life and world. Our world is increasingly struggling with wars, violence, and inhumane acts—be they human-to human, human-to-environment, or human-to-nature.

In spite of an evolved cosmology for all disciplines today, including physics and basic sciences and other scientific fields, we still often find ourselves locked in outdated thinking within a separatist-material-physical world ontology and an outer-worldview as our starting point. Caring Science, in contrast, has as its starting point a relational ontology that honors the fact that we are all connected and Belong to

Source—the universal spirit field of infinity (Levinas 1969)—before and after the human plane of worldly experiences. Caring Science makes more explicit that unity and connectedness exist among all things in the great circle of life: change, illness, suffering, death, and rebirth. A Caring Science orientation moves humanity closer to a moral community, closer to peaceful relationships with self–other communities–nations, states, other worlds, and time.

BASIC ASSUMPTIONS OF CARING SCIENCE (ADAPTED WITH MINOR MODIFICATIONS FROM WATSON 1979:8–9)

- Caring Science is the essence of nursing and the foundational disciplinary core of the profession.

- Caring can be most effectively demonstrated and practiced interpersonally; however, caring consciousness can be communicated beyond/transcends time, space, and physicality (Watson 2002a).

- The intersubjective human-to-human processes and connections keep alive a common sense of humanity; they teach us how to be human by identifying ourselves with others, whereby the humanity of one is reflected in the other (Watson 1985:33).

- Caring consists of Carative Factors/*Caritas Processes* that facilitate healing, honor wholeness, and contribute to the evolution of humanity.

- Effective Caring promotes healing, health, individual/family growth and a sense of wholeness, forgiveness, evolved consciousness, and inner peace that transcends the crisis and fear of disease, diagnosis, illness, traumas, life changes, and so on.

- Caring responses accept a person not only as he or she is now but as what he or she may become/is Becoming.

- A Caring relationship is one that invites emergence of human spirit, opening to authentic potential, being authentically present, allowing the person to explore options—choosing the best action for self for "being-in-right relation" at any given point in time.

- Caring is more "healthogenic" than curing.

- Caring Science is complementary to Curing Science.

- The practice of Caring is central to nursing. Its social, moral, and scientific contributions lie in its professional commitment to the values, ethics, and ideals of Caring Science in theory, practice, and research.

PREMISES OF CARING SCIENCE
(ADAPTED FROM WATSON 2005:218–219)

- Knowledge of Caring cannot be assumed; it is an epistemic-ethical-theoretical endeavor that requires ongoing explication and development.

- Caring Science is grounded in a relational, ethical ontology of unity within the universe that informs the epistemology, methodology, pedagogy, and praxis of caring in nursing and related fields.

- Caring Science embraces epistemological pluralism, seeking to understand the intersection and underdeveloped connections between the arts and humanities and the clinical sciences.

- Caring Science embraces all ways of knowing/being/doing: ethical, intuitive, personal, empirical, aesthetic, and even spiritual/metaphysical ways of knowing and Being.

- Caring Science inquiry encompasses methodological pluralism, whereby the method flows from the phenomenon of concern—diverse forms of inquiry seek to unify ontological, philosophical, ethical, and theoretical views while incorporating empirics and technology.

- Caring (and nursing) has existed in every society. Every society has had some people who have cared for others. A caring attitude is *not* transmitted from generation to generation by genes. It is transmitted by the culture of a society. The culture of nursing, in this instance the discipline and profession of nursing, has a vital social-scientific role in advancing, sustaining, and preserving human caring as a way of fulfilling its mission to society and broader humanity.

WORKING DEFINITION OF CARING SCIENCE (EXTRACTED/MODIFIED FROM WATSON 2004A; WATSON AND SMITH 2002)

Caring Science is an evolving philosophical-ethical-epistemic field of study, grounded in the discipline of nursing and informed by related fields. Caring is considered as one central feature within the meta-paradigm of nursing knowledge and practice. Caring Science is informed by an ethical-moral-spiritual stance that encompasses a humanitarian, human science orientation to human caring processes, phenomena, and experiences. It is located within a worldview that is non-dualistic, relational, and unified, wherein there is a connectedness to All: the universal field of Infinity: Cosmic LOVE. This worldview is sometimes referred to as

- A unitary transformative paradigm (Newman, Sime, and Corcoran-Perry 1991; Watson 1999)
- Nonlocal consciousness (Dossey 1991)
- Era III medicine/nursing (Dossey 1991, 1993; Watson 1999).

Caring Science within this worldview intersects with the arts and humanities and related fields of study and practice.

CARING: SCIENCE-ARTS-HUMANITIES

To understand nursing as a discipline and a distinct field of study is to honor it within a context of art, the humanities, and expanding views of science. As a distinct discipline, it is necessary to acknowledge that nursing and Caring reside within a humanitarian as well as a scientific matrix; thus, there is an intersection among the arts, humanities, philosophy, science, and technology. The discipline encompasses a broad worldview that honors evolving humanity and an evolving universe that is full of wonder and unknowns as well as known set expectations about our world.

Just as the profession may detour at times from its disciplinary heritage, so too we often forget that an equal need exists for humanistic-aesthetic views of a similar phenomenon. Humanities and the arts seek to answer different questions than science does. It continues to be important to understand the essential characteristics they all bring and the ways in which they are similar and different and in which they also converge.

For example, conventional science is concerned with order, prediction, control, methods, generalizations, detachment, objectivity, and so forth. The three classical assumptions that have shaped modern conventional science are *objectivism, positivism, and reductionism* (Harman 1990–1991; Watson 2005). Science in this context cannot answer certain questions about humanity, about caring and what it means to be human. Science generally is not concerned with specific individual responses but more with prediction and generalizations about anonymous others. It cannot be expected or called upon to keep alive a sense of common humanity (Watson 1979:4). It does not offer insights into depth of human experiences such as pain, joy, suffering, fear, forgiveness, love, and so on. Such in-depth exploration of humanity is expressed and pondered through study of philosophy, drama, the arts, film, literature, humanistic studies in the liberal arts, humanities proper, and so on. This perspective is learned through self-knowledge, self-discovery, and shared human experiences, combined with the study of human emotions and relations that mirror our shared humanity.

In spite of inherent differences between science and the humanities, both fields and, in fact, all fields of study are changing, expanding, growing into new dynamic intersections between and among each other. There is a convergence between and among art, science, and spirituality; this convergence is becoming more prevalent among emerging models of mind-body-spirit medicine, so-called complementary-alternative-integrative medicine, and new understandings of the physics of science, energy medicine, spirituality and healing, and so forth.

The intersections between art and science help reveal what is beyond the confines and contingencies of the visible world, to "see" that which is deeper, glimpsing the human spirit, the human soul, its beauty and loveliness, whatever its shape or form (Housden 2005:3). As Housden put it, art helps our eyes see more than they usually do: about life in general but also about ourselves. The same can be said for the humanities, drama, and also science, opening up a new horizon of meaning and possibilities. However, art helps us "to bear witness to eternal joy, suffering, pain and struggle of our own human soul and to feel the poignant, bittersweet reality of our physical mortality" (Housden 2005:3). In their own ways, art and science remind us that we are "both finite and infinite and everything in between" (Housden

2005:10–11). In considering Caring Science, art, the humanities, and the beauty of science and life itself all come into play. When one is engaged in human caring and healing, one cannot ignore the element of aesthetics and beauty and the spiritual domain of life's journey.

In Emerson's words: "This element [beauty] I call an ultimate end. No reason can be asked or given why the soul seeks beauty. Beauty in its largest and most profound sense is one expression of the universe" (Emerson 1982:48). In this sense, then, art transforms us and helps us to see our everyday world differently, in that arts move us into a space where we can create visions of other ways of Being/doing/knowing and ask what it might signify to realize them (Greene 1991). It is this engagement in art and a sense of beauty that gives rise to wonder, to questioning, and to pondering our Being.

The art and science of caring-healing is emerging in mainstream medicine and nursing, as the public has a hunger for the intersection among art, science, beauty, and spiritual dimensions of the healing arts and health and also has a greater sense of self-knowledge, self-control, and well-being. As Kandinsky (1977) understood it, "the spiritual resides in art" (just as Emerson viewed nature as spirit); perhaps they are one and the same, tapping into the human spirit of humanity and the universal source of infinity in which we dwell.

In any event, in nursing and caring-healing work, we draw upon healing arts in a more expanded way that integrates science, art, beauty, and spirituality. These are manifest in unlimited potential for areas such as visual arts, music, sound, aroma, dance, movement, theater, drama, storytelling, design, psycho-architecture/sacred healing architecture, and a variety of tactile-touch and noncontact, energetic modalities.

Diverse categories of healing arts are emerging. At least four types have been identified:

- Art intended to directly heal, using symbols, images that calm and center.
- Art created by artists to facilitate their own healing; for example, autobiographical art, representational art depicting incidences of treatment, illness, change.

- Art about specific aspects of the healing process—pain, loss, body image changes, loss, grief, death, as well as hope, change, joy, insights, and so forth.

- Artist-designed psycho-architecture; healing spaces/healing architecture—this art/architecture makes a conscious, intentional, even a technical, precise scientific effort to integrate symbol, myth, archetype, mystery, and legend into architectural and environmental themes. Such art can be considered "ontological design," an integration of sacred geometry into architectural structures so humans can "be" and feel differently as a way of experiencing self-in-harmony, with the sacred universal field of life's energy for healing, wholeness, alignment, and so on. (Lafo, Capasso, and Roberts 1994:9)

Caring Science seeks to combine science with the humanities and arts. Caring Science is not neutral with respect to human values, goals, subjective individual perceptions, and meanings. It is not detached from human emotions and their diverse expressions, be they culturally bound or individually revealed.

The discipline of nursing—guided by a Caring Science orientation—seeks to study, research, explore, identify, describe, express, and question the relation and intersection between and among the ethical, ontological, epistemological, methodological, pedagogical, and praxis aspects of nursing, including health policies and administrative practices. Thus, a Caring Science orientation seeks congruence between and among clinical nursing science, humanities, the arts, and the human subject matter and phenomena of caring knowledge and practices.

ONTOLOGICAL "COMPETENCIES": CARING LITERACY*

In moving from a discussion of art, beauty, the humanities, and science, perhaps there is more awareness of the connection between

---

* The movement from the notion of "ontological competencies" to the concept of "Caring Literacy" is influenced by Joan Boyce, Victoria University, British Columbia, PhD dissertation: Nurses Making Caring Work: A Closet Drama, and the discussion during her PhD final examination, June 2007.

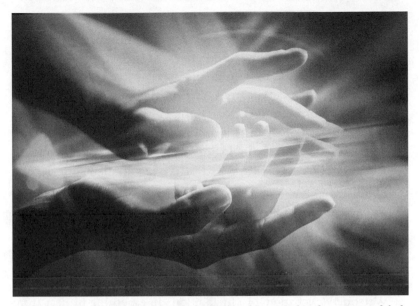

Figure 5. Hands of light and love—the basis of healing in midst of institutional darkness. Hans Neleman/Getty Images.

this integrated way of thinking about Caring Science and Human Artistry. Such notions translate into what I have previously referred to as *"Ontological Competencies,"* reframed as *"Caring Literacy,"* or *"Caritas Literacy."*

While the meaning of literacy is associated with the abilities to read and write, the notion of having fluency in caring at both personal and professional levels introduces new meaning to deepen our ways of attending to and cultivating how to *Be-deeply Human/humane* and *Be-Caring* and Having a Healing presence. This form of *Being* is a form of human literacy, human artistry.

Such literacy includes an evolved and continually evolving emotional heart intelligence, consciousness, and intentionality and level of sensitivity and efficacy, followed by a continuing lifelong process and journey of self-growth and self-awareness. Such an awakening of one's being and abilities cultivates skills and awareness of holding, conveying, and practicing communicating thoughts of caring, loving, kindness, equanimity, and so on as part of one's professional Being.

This level of evolved Being/Ontological presence is now ethically required for any professional engaged in caring-healing. Perhaps this requirement was and has always been present in the tradition of healing professions, but somewhere along the way professional education and practices took a detour from the very foundation of our shared humanity. A return to a focus on Ontological Competencies, within the evolved notion of Caring Literacy, seems essential to balance and carry out the pervasive technological competencies, helping to make these skills and forms of Being part of the requirements for nursing education and practice.

EXAMPLES OF (ONTOLOGICAL) CARING LITERACY

I have only begun to identify some of these so-called Ontological Competencies for cultivating Caring Literacy (Watson 1999). (For more exploration of these ideas within the context of Nightingale, see Watson 1999:chapter 14.) In addition, an emerging project from the International Caritas Consortium (ICC) is focused on Caring Literacy and *Caritas* Literacy, seeking more and more specificity in the knowledge, skills, and ways of being to manifest such literacy. A working document is found in the Addenda as well as on the Web site www.caritasconsortium.org.*

In the meantime, I have identified the following general guideline dimensions as examples of "ontological competencies" that facilitate Caring Literacy. These directions have emerged from my work over

---

* A subgroup from the ICC has a current, ongoing working draft of Caring/ *Caritas* Literacy. It is found in Addendum III.

This latest ICC document on Caritas Literacy is based on meetings, dialogue, and previous work among the subgroup members: J. D'Alfonso, Scottsdale Health, Scottsdale, Arizona; J. Duffy, The Catholic University of America, Washington, D.C.; Gene Rigotti, InovaHealth, Fairfax, Virginia; J. Watson, University of Colorado–Denver and Health Sciences, Denver, Colorado; and Terri Woodward, The Children's Hospital, Denver, Colorado. The items marked with a check on this document represent items on the Caring Assessment Tool ©-Version IV (Duffy, Hoskins, and Seifert 2007).

the past decade or so and need to continue to unfold with more specificity—something related to the ICC project—ultimately leading to better documentation and assessment of Caring/*Caritas*.

I invite readers to identify the ontological-literacy processes they bring to their caring-healing practice and to continue to contribute to more specificity so these practices can be taught, documented, researched, and practiced.

WATSON'S *CARITAS* LITERACY DIMENSIONS: A WORK IN PROGRESS

- Cultivate Caring consciousness and intentionality as a starting point
- Ability to "Center"—quiet down, pause before entering patient's room or be still in the presence of the other
- Ability to "read the field" when entering into the life space or field of another
- Ability to *Be present—Be with* other as well as *Do for* other
- Accurately identify and address person by name
- Maintain eye contact as appropriate for person/cultural meaning and sensitivity
- Ability to ground self and other for comforting, soothing, calming acts
- Accurately detect other's feelings
- Stay within the other's frame of reference
- Invite and authentically listen to the inner meaning, the subjective story of other
- Authentically listen/hear behind the words
- Hold other with an attitude of unconditional loving-kindness, equanimity, dignity, and regard
- Ability to be with "silence," waiting for other to reflect before responding to questions, allowing other's inner thoughts to emerge
- Respond to the other's feelings and mood verbally and nonverbally, with authentic affective congruence

- Cultivate and create meaningful caring-healing rituals: translate conventional nursing tasks into purposive healing acts
  - For example, hand washing as purification, cleansing psychically as well as physically; use as opportunity to "center," release, and bless patient/situation while preparing oneself to enter into next moment
  - Incorporate, translate, and expand nursing skills/tasks into nursing arts/caring-healing modalities: for example, intentional use of music-sound, touch, aroma, visual-aesthetic-beauty, energetic approaches, and so on
  - Carry out conventional nursing tasks and procedures, such as basic needs and physical care acts, as intentional, reverential, respectful caring-healing arts
  - Cultivate own practices for spiritual growth and evolution of higher/deeper consciousness
  - Others—yet to be identified (see www.caritasconsortium.org).

We need to continue to explore models for cultivating Caring Literacy and skill in attending to our human presence in "Being-in-caring-healing-relationships." These directions incorporate aspects of caring such as silence, song, music, poetry, physical and nonphysical touch, centering practices of "presencing"; the use of art, nonverbal expressive forms, spirit-energy-filled conscious affirmations; holding intentions of wholeness, calmness, healing, and so on.

Within this framework of Caring Literacy, it is important to realize that the nurse is not only *in* the environment, able to make significant changes in ways of Being/doing/knowing in the physical environment, but that the *nurse IS the environment* (Quinn 1992; Watson 2005). Thus, the nurse is invited to engage in significant insight into the *Nurse-Self* as an energetic-vibrational field of consciousness and intentionality (Quinn 1992), affecting the entire environment for better or for worse. The nurse's (caring-loving) consciousness radiates higher vibrational effects. A nurse without an informed, "literate" caring consciousness can actually be "biocidic"—that is, toxic, life destroying, and destructive to the experience of others (Halldorsdottir 1991). On the other hand, a nurse who is cultivating ontological competencies in Caring Literacy is more likely to be "biogenic"—that is, life giving and life receiving for self and other and thereby more likely to engage in and experience a transpersonal caring-healing moment. As the nurse cultivates these ontological literate abilities and sensitivities of caring, there is an invitation to open to inner healing processes that expand to infinite new possibilities.

Ontological–Caring Literacy directions serve only as examples of the intersection between technological competencies and emotional-intellectual literacy of human caring skills of *Being-Caring*. Such exploration into the literacy of caring incorporates the ethical, philosophical, and theoretical foundations of professional caring-healing. This view of Caring Literacy serves as core knowledge that leads directly back to the original Carative Factors and the evolution toward *Caritas Consciousness* and *Caritas Processes*. These evolved concepts are presented in Chapter 2.

CHAPTER TWO

CARATIVE FACTORS / *CARITAS PROCESSES:*

Original and Evolved Core for Professional Nursing

The background on my major books on Caring Theory, Philosophy, and Caring Science helps us see the evolution of my original work. This revised, updated edition builds upon the primary source material from the 1979 text and its evolution from what is known as the ten Carative Factors (CFs) toward ten *Caritas Processes* (CPs). Likewise, this revision incorporates ideas from my previous published works, summarized and developed as background in Section I.

Table 2.1 includes the original 1979 Carative Factors (with minor edits from the 1985 book). The original ten Carative Factors, juxtaposed against the emerging *Caritas Processes,* are summarized in Table 2.2.

CORE ASPECTS THEORY OF HUMAN CARING

- Relational Caring as ethical-moral-philosophical values-guided foundation

Table 2.1 Original Ten Carative Factors, Original (1979) Text

1. Formation of a humanistic-altruistic system of values
2. Instillation of faith-hope
3. Cultivation of sensitivity to oneself and others
4. Development of a helping-trusting relationship
5. Promotion and acceptance of the expression of positive and negative feelings
6. Systematic use of the scientific problem-solving method for decision making (refined in 1985 as use of creative problem-solving caring process)
7. Promotion of interpersonal teaching-learning
8. Provision for a supportive, protective, and (or) corrective mental, physical, sociocultural, and spiritual environment
9. Assistance with gratification of human needs
10. Allowance for existential-phenomenological forces (refined in 1985 as existential-phenomenological spiritual dimensions)

Source: J. Watson (1979). *Nursing: The Philosophy and Science of Caring*. Boston: Little, Brown, 9–10.

- Caring core: Ten Carative Factors / *Caritas Processes*
- Transpersonal *Caring Moment–Caring Field*
- Caring as consciousness—energy-intentionality–human presence
- Caring-Healing modalities.

The ten original Carative Factors remain the timeless structural core of the theory while allowing for their evolving emergence into more fluid aspects of the model captured by the ten *Caritas Processes*.

In introducing the original concept of Carative Factors as the core for a nursing philosophy and science, I was offering a theoretical counterpoint to the notion of Curative, so dominant in medical science. Thus, the Carative Factors provided a framework to hold the discipline and profession of nursing; they were informed by a deeper vision and ethical commitment to the human dimensions of caring in nursing—the art and human science context. I was seeking to address those aspects of professional nursing that transcended medical diagnosis, disease, setting, limited and changing knowledge, and the technological emphasis on very specialized phenomena.

I was asking, What remains as core? My response in 1979 was "The Ten Carative Factors" (embellished in 2007 by the philosophical-ethical value of *Caritas-loving* consciousness).

Table 2.2 Original Carative Factors and Evolved *Caritas Processes*

Carative Factors 1979	*Caritas Processes* 2002–2007
1. Humanistic-altruistic values	1. Practicing loving-kindness and equanimity for self and other
2. Instilling/enabling faith and hope	2. Being authentically present; enabling/sustaining/honoring deep belief system and subjective world of self/other
3. Cultivating sensitivity to oneself and other	3. Cultivating one's own spiritual practices; deepening self-awareness, going beyond "ego-self"
4. Developing a helping-trusting, human caring relationship	4. Developing and sustaining a helping-trusting, authentic caring relationship
5. Promoting and accepting expression of positive and negative feelings	5. Being present to, and supportive of, the expression of positive and negative feelings as a connection with deeper spirit of self and the one-being-cared-for
6. Systematic use of scientific (creative) problem-solving caring process	6. Creative use of self and all ways of knowing/being/doing as part of the caring process (engaging in artistry of caring-healing practices)
7. Promoting transpersonal teaching-learning	7. Engaging in genuine teaching-learning experiences within context of caring relationship—attend to whole person and subjective meaning; attempt to stay within other's frame of reference (evolve toward "coaching" role vs. conventional imparting of information)
8. Providing for a supportive, protective, and/or corrective mental, social, spiritual environment	8. Creating healing environment at all levels (physical, nonphysical, subtle environment of energy and consciousness whereby wholeness, beauty, comfort, dignity, and peace are potentiated (Being/Becoming the environment)
9. Assisting with gratification of human needs	9. Reverentially and respectfully assisting with basic needs; holding an intentional, caring consciousness of touching and working with the embodied spirit of another, honoring unity of Being; allowing for spirit-filled connection
10. Allowing for existential-phenomenological dimensions	10. Opening and attending to spiritual, mysterious, unknown existential dimensions of life-death-suffering; *"allowing for a miracle"**

* Idea courtesy Resurrection Health, Chicago.
Sources: J. Watson (1979). *Nursing: The Philosophy and Science of Caring.* Boston: Little, Brown; www.uchsc.edu/nursing/caring.

The CFs were identified as the essential core of professional nursing practice, in contrast to what I called the "trim," that which is constantly changing and cannot be the content or the criteria with which to describe, identify, and sustain professional nursing and its timeless disciplinary stance with respect to caring in society.

As indicated in the original (1979) work, "carative" was a word I made up to serve as a counterpoint to the "curative" orientation of medical science. I identified these ten factors as the core activities and orientations a professional nurse uses in the delivery of care. They are the common and necessary professional practices that sustain and reveal nursing as a distinct (caring) profession, not as comprising a group of technicians. Nurses apply the CFs constantly but are not aware of them, nor have they necessarily named them. Thus, nurses generally are not conscious of their own phenomena; they do not have the language to identify, chart, and communicate systematically and so on. This is a result of both a lack of awareness and terminology of caring and of recognized knowledge of those everyday practices that define their work. Without an awareness, additional education, and advancement of professional caring in nursing, these factors are likely to occur in an ad hoc, rather than a systematic, fashion.

Nurses will not be aware or realize the importance of using them/ *Becoming* them to guide their professional caring practices. Further, without a context to hold these practices, nurses have often devalued their caring work, taking it for granted, without a common language to "see," articulate, act on, reinforce, and advance that work.

If nurses are committed to a model of professional caring-healing, going beyond conventional medicalized-clinical routines and industrial product-line views of nursing (and humanity), yet do not have a theoretical guide to honor, frame, discuss, develop, and advance their profession, a demoralized experience and despair set in over time (Swanson 1999). If this continues, there is little hope for the survival of professional nursing and its caring-healing practices. Likewise, without furthering this work, there is little to no hope for advancement of Caring Science as the disciplinary foundation for nursing (and other health sciences), little hope for a foundation that guides and contains the values, ethics, moral foundation, and philosophical directions for caring for human beings. Without honoring and attending to Caring Science knowledge and practices, nursing will not be fulfilling its scientific, ethical, professional covenant with its public or even with itself.

MOVING FROM CARATIVE TO *CARITAS*

From an academic standpoint related to knowledge development and theory evolution, one can consider that I used the technical process of concept derivation (Walker and Avant 2005) and extension in transposing and redefining Carative Factors to *Caritas Processes*. That is, in working within the original field of Nursing and Carative thinking, I sought to redefine Carative from the parent field, Nursing, to the new field of Caring Science with its explicit ethic, worldview, and so on.

Thus, once the Carative concept was transposed from nursing per se to Caring Science, *Caritas/Caritas Processes* emerged as a more meaningful concept, generating new connections between Caring and Love. The broader field of Caring Science and its expanded cosmology of unity, belonging, and infinity of the universal field of Love allowed for a more meaningful redefinition for the phenomenon of *Caritas Nursing* to result. As the transposition from Carative Nursing to *Caritas* Caring Science occurred, a new vocabulary for an ontological phenomenon was revealed, allowing for new ways of thinking about caring and inviting a new image, even a metaphor, of caring-healing practices to develop. Further, the new notion of *Caritas* offers a new vocabulary/phenomenon for an area of inquiry, leading to additional theorizing and knowledge development at the disciplinary level of nursing and Caring Science.

Table 2.3 is a visual depiction of the process of Concept derivation for extending the theory of human caring from Carative nursing to *Caritas* within a Caring Science context.

While each of the original Carative Factors has been transposed and extended into the new language of *Caritas*, several core principles are the most essential with respect to a change in consciousness. These five cultivated areas of *Caritas* are those that help distinguish the core differences between the notions of Carative and *Caritas*.

Table 2.3 Visual Representation of Concept Derivation and Extension from Carative Nursing to *Caritas Processes* in Caring Science

Concept I:	*Transposed to*	Concept I:	*Redefined*	Concept II:
Carative Factors		Carative		Field II:
Field I: Nursing		New Field II:		*Caritas Processes*
		Caring Science		in Caring Science

CORE PRINCIPLES/PRACTICES: FROM CARATIVE TO *CARITAS*

- Practice of loving-kindness and equanimity
- Authentic presence: enabling deep belief of other
- Cultivation of one's own spiritual practice—beyond ego
- "Being" the caring-healing environment
- Allowing for miracles.

In moving from the concept of Carative to *Caritas,* I am overtly evoking Love and Caring to merge into an expanded paradigm for the future. Such a perspective ironically places nursing in its most mature paradigm while reconnecting with the heritage and foundation of Nightingale. With *Caritas* incorporated more explicitly, it locates the theory within an ethical and ontological context as the starting point for considering not only its science but also its societal mission for humanity. This direction makes a more formal connection between caring and healing and the evolved human consciousness. The background for this work is available in Watson (2004a).

EMERGENCE OF *CARITAS NURSING* AND THE *CARITAS NURSE*

My evolution toward *Caritas Processes* is intended to offer a more fluid language for understanding a deeper, more comprehensive level of the work, as well as guidance toward how to enter into, interpret, sustain, and inquire about the intention and consciousness behind the original Carative Factors. Moreover, *Caritas* captures a deeper phenomenon, a new image that intersects professional-personal practices while opening up a new field of inquiry for nursing and Caring Science.

However, as one steps into this new work, it is important to consider both the original CFs and the evolved CPs holographically, in that the whole is in any and every part. So all the factors/processes are simultaneously present; they are either foreground or background when practicing within a professional caring model. Further, the consciousness/intentionality of caring-healing and wholeness is held by the nurse as part of his or her presence in the moment.

What is emerging throughout this shift to *Caritas Processes* is an acknowledgment of a deeper form of nursing: *Caritas Nursing and the Caritas Nurse*. As the work evolves and as each nurse evolves, we learn throughout this book that the more evolved practitioner (working from the higher/deeper dimensions of humanity and evolving consciousness) can be identified as a *Caritas Nurse*, or one who is practicing or at least cultivating the practices of *Caritas Nursing*. Another way to identify a *Caritas Nurse* is as one who is working from a human-to-human connection—working from an open, intelligent heart center* rather than the ego-center. This caring consciousness orientation informs the professional actions and relationships of a *Caritas Nurse*, even while she or he is engaged in the required routine or dramatic, practical-technical world of clinical practices.

For example, in considering CF 1: Humanistic, altruistic value systems, one may wonder what is behind and underneath such a value system that allows it to manifest professionally in one's actions. How is such a value system to be cultivated and sustained for professional caring practices? What personal practices can prepare one for entering into and manifesting this value system throughout one's career?

My response is that this value system comes to life when one cultivates the ongoing practice of Loving-Kindness and Equanimity, a form of cultivated mindfulness awareness/meditation, a practice that opens and awakens the compassionate, forgiving love of the heart center. This preparation can take the form of daily practice of offering gratitude, of connecting with nature; the practice of silence, journaling, prayer; asking for guidance to be there for another when needed; developing

---

* More on the open heart focus is found in the discussion of chakra systems in Chapter 18. As a prelude, *Caritas Nursing* requires cultivation of higher, deeper consciousness, working more and more to awaken the heart-centered chakra upward to the crown chakra in bringing one's full and open self into any caring occasion.

a practice of forgiveness, silently citing positive affirmations, opening to blessings in the midst of difficulties, whereby one's consciousness is expanded through all these practices. These are only some examples of how to enter into and sustain this professional ethic of altruism and loving-kindness. This work is related not only to caring but also to the health and healing of practitioner as well as patient.

If "health is expanded consciousness," as Newman posits (Newman 1994), then what is the highest level of consciousness? *It is Love* in the fullest universal, cosmic sense. What is the greatest source of Healing? It, too, is Love. So, in cultivating the practice of loving-kindness toward self and other, one is opening his or her heart; one is heightened to give and receive, to be present to what is presenting itself in one's life; to open to exercising and receiving grace, mercy, forgiveness, and so on. Thus, one can better appreciate the gifts of giving and receiving, being there for another person to offer presence, loving consciousness, and informed moral caring actions in the midst of suffering, despair, love, hate, illness, sorrow, questions, trauma, unknowns, fears, hopes, and so on. In this personal/professional caring work, one cultivates an acceptance, a level of humility, before the mystery of it all—opening to it with equanimity, compassion, and mercy as part of the human condition. This level of consciousness with which to enter and sustain professional caring in nursing, while honoring our deep humanity, is founded on a very different model than conventional nursing and medicine.

This mode of *Caritas* thinking invites a total transformation of self and systems. In this model of Caring Science, the changes occur not from the outer focus on systems but from that deep inner place within the creativity of the human spirit. Here is where the deep humanity, the individual heart and consciousness of practitioners, evolves and connects with the ultimate source of all true re-formation/transformation.

While the original Carative Factors remain relevant and accessible for first-level concrete entry into the work, once one grows with the ideas and their evolution, it is hoped that one moves more fully into a knowing that is behind the original material and enters a more profound level of insight, personal/professional growth, understanding, and wisdom. At the same time, the shift allows for nurses and nursing to evolve toward accessing a more fluid, expressive language for comprehending and articulating the deeper meaning behind the original factors.

CHAPTER THREE

CARITAS PROCESSES: *Extension of Carative Factors*

CARING AND LOVE

One day, after we have mastered the winds and the waves, gravity and the tides, we will harness for God the energies of love.

TEILHARD DE CHARDIN

Caritas comes from the Latin word meaning to cherish, to appreciate, to give special, if not loving, attention to. It represents charity and compassion, generosity of spirit. It connotes something very fine, indeed, something precious that needs to be cultivated and sustained.

Caritas is closely related to the word "Carative" from my original (1979) text on Caring Science. However, now, using the terms *Caritas* and *Caritas Processes*, I invoke intentionally the *"L" word: Love*, which makes explicit the connection between caring and love, Love in its fullest universal infinite sense developed in the philosophy of Levinas (1969) and explored in my 2005 text *Caring Science as Sacred Science.*

Bringing Love and Caring together this way invites a form of deep transpersonal caring. The relationship between Love and Caring creates an opening/alignment and access for inner healing for self and others. While health may be considered to represent expanding consciousness, Love is the highest level of consciousness and the greatest source of all healing in the world. This connection with Love as a source for healing extends from the individual self to nature and the larger universe, which is evolving and unfolding. This cosmology and worldview of Caring and Love—*Caritas*—is both grounded and metaphysical; it is immanent and transcendent with the co-evolving human in the universe (Watson 1999, 2004a).

It is when we include and bring together Caring and Love in our work and our lives that we discover and affirm that nursing, like teaching, is more than a job. It is a life-giving and life-receiving career for a lifetime of growth and learning. It is maturing in an awakening and an awareness that nursing has much more to offer humankind than simply being an extension of an outdated model of medicine and medical-techno-cure science. Nursing helps sustain human dignity and humanity itself while contributing to the evolution of human consciousness, helping to move toward a more humane and caring moral community and civilization.

As nursing more publicly and professionally asserts these positions from a Caring Science context for its theories, ethics, and practices, we are invited to relocate ourselves and our profession away from a dominant medical science mind-set. Further, we are asked to reconnect nursing's disciplinary source to its noble heritage, within both an ancient and an emerging cosmology—a cosmology that invites and welcomes the energy of universal caring and love back into our lives and world. Such thinking calls forth a sense of reverence and sacredness with regard to our work, our lives, and all living things. It incorporates art, science, and spirituality as they are being redefined.

As we enter into a maturing of Caring Science and evolved *Caritas Processes* as a professional-theoretical map and guide, we are simultaneously challenged to relocate ourselves in these emerging ideals and ideas and question for ourselves how this work speaks to us as a discipline and a practice profession. Each person is asked, invited, if not enticed, to examine, explore, challenge, and question for self and for the profession the critical intersections between the personal and the professional.

This revised work calls each of us into our deepest self to give new meaning to our lives and work, to explore how our unique gifts, talents, and skills can be translated into compassionate human caring–healing service for self and others and even the planet Earth. It is hoped that at some level this work will help us all, in the caring-healing professions, to remember who we are and why we have come here to do this work in the world.

VALUE ASSUMPTIONS OF *CARITAS*
(ADAPTED FROM WATSON 1985:32)

- Caring and Love are the most universal, tremendous, and mysterious cosmic forces; they comprise the primal and universal source of energy.

- Often this wisdom is overlooked, or we forget, even though we know people need each other in loving and caring ways.

- If our humanity is to survive and if we are to evolve toward a more loving, caring, deeply human and humane, moral community and civilization, we must sustain love and caring in our life, our work, our world.

- Since nursing is a caring profession, its ability to sustain its caring ideals, ethics, and philosophy for professional practices will affect the human development of civilization and nursing's mission in society.

- As a beginning, we have to learn how to offer caring, love, forgiveness, compassion, and mercy to ourselves before we can offer authentic caring and love to others.

- We have to treat ourselves with loving-kindness and equanimity, gentleness and dignity before we can accept, respect, and care for others within a professional caring-healing model.

- Nursing has always held a caring stance with respect to others and their health-illness concerns.

- Knowledgeable, informed, ethical caring is the essence of professional nursing values, commitments, and competent actions; it is the most central and unifying source to sustain its covenant to society and ensure its survival.

- Preservation and advancement of Caring Science values, knowledge, theories, philosophies, ethics, and clinical practices, within a context of an expanding *Caritas* cosmology, are ontological, epistemological, and clinical endeavors; these endeavors are the source and foundation for sustaining and advancing the discipline and profession.

Return to Love as the Basis for *Caritas Consciousness* and Gratitude Toward Self-Others

In a world like ours, where death is increasingly drained of meaning, individual authenticity lies in what we can find that is worth living for. And the only thing worth living for is love. Love for one another. Love for ourselves. Love of our work. Love of our destiny, whatever it may be. Love for our difficulties. Love of life. The love that could free us from the mysterious cycles of suffering. The love that releases us from our self-imprisonment, from our bitterness, our greed, our madness-engendering competitiveness. The love that can make us breathe again. Love a great and beautiful cause, a wonderful vision. A great love for another, or for the future. The love that reconciles us to ourselves, to our simple joys, and to our undiscovered repletion. A creative love. A love touched with the sublime. (Okri 1997:56–57)

CARITAS PROCESS—CULTIVATING THE PRACTICE OF LOVING-KINDNESS AND EQUANIMITY TOWARD SELF AND OTHER AS FOUNDATIONAL TO *CARITAS CONSCIOUSNESS*

When love moves through us it inspires all we do.
Love and compassion must begin with kindness toward ourselves.
One of the greatest blocks to loving kindness is our own sense of unworthiness.

KORNFIELD (2002:95, 101, 100)

The Carative Factor: Formation of Humanistic-Altruistic Values system continues to lay the foundation as a starting point for Caring Science.

As a given, caring must be grounded within a set of universal human values—kindness, concern, and love of self and others. As one matures into a professional model that focuses on caring-healing and health in its broadest and deepest dimensions, such as the timeless mission of nursing, one must cultivate an awareness and intentionality to sustain such a guiding vision for one's life and work. This factor in its original and evolved sense honors the gift of being able to give and receive with a capacity to love and appreciate all of life's diversity and its individuality with each person. Such a system helps us to tolerate difference and view others through their subjective worldview rather than ours alone.

Regardless of whether one is conscious of one's own philosophy and value system, it is affecting the encounters, relationships, and moments we have with our self and others. These humanistic-altruistic values can be developed through a variety of life experiences: early childhood, exposure to different languages and cultures, history, as well as film, drama, art, literature, and other creative expressions of humanity and personal growth experiences.

These emotions of love, kindness, gentleness, compassion, equanimity, and so on are intrinsic to all humans. These emotions and experiences are the essence of what makes us human and what deepens our humanity and our connection with the human spirit. This awareness is what connects us with the "Source" from which we draw our sacred breath for life itself. It is here where we access our energy and creativity for living and being; it is here, in this model, that we yield to that which is greater than our individual ego-self, reminding us that we belong to the universe of humanity and all living things.

For this original Carative Factor (CF) to evolve and mature in its manifestation, we are now called, invited, and challenged to take it to a deeper level in our maturity, our awareness, our experiences and expressions. This is a path of deepening who and what we are that prepares us for a lifelong commitment to caring-healing and compassionate human service. Thus, the evolution/extension of the original CF has been both sustained and transcended. The original CFs and evolved *Caritas Processes* are considered the bedrock and most basic foundation for preparing practitioners to engage in and practice the Philosophy, Science, (and ethic) of Caring.

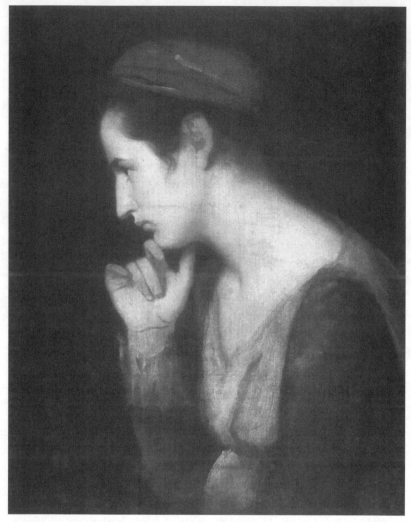

Figure 6. Contemplation, *by George Romney. Collection, The Denver Art Museum.*

PART III

From *Carative Factors to* Caritas Processes

CHAPTER FOUR

From **CARATIVE FACTOR 1:** *Humanistic-Altruistic*
System of Values
to **CARITAS PROCESS 1:** *Cultivating the Practice of*
Loving-Kindness and Equanimity Toward Self and Other as
Foundational to Caritas Consciousness

Preparing for any worthwhile endeavor requires the cultivation of skills to engage in doing the chosen work. One cannot enter into and sustain *Caritas* practices for caring-healing without being personally prepared. It is ironic that nursing education and practice require so much knowledge and skill to *do* the job, but very little effort is directed toward developing how to *Be* while doing the real work of the job. Nurses often become pained and worn down by trying to always care, give, and be there for others without attending to the loving care needed for self. This model invites, if not requires, nurses to attend to self-caring and practices that assist in their own evolution of consciousness for more fulfillment in their life and work.

In this way of thinking, nurses can be models and living exemplars by beginning to openly stand for what people have not been doing— that is, articulating, Becoming-Being-Living the work that needs to be done for this planet and humanity at this point in human history (Young personal communication, 2006).

We can become part of a global vision of health and human transformation to help purify the toxins and poisons; the negativity of violence, abuse, war; the noncaring and disregard for the human-environment-universe connection for self and all living things.

Perhaps the new role for *Caritas Nursing* is to transform the vision of human health and healing by engaging in service to self and society at a different level by creating the "energetic field of *Caritas*" through both overt and subtle practices that transmit and affect the field of the whole.

Nurses can do this one by one and become part of creating a deeper level of humanity by transforming fundamentally what happens in a given moment, in a given situation, by experimenting with *Being-the-Caritas-Field*. This is the truly deep, noble work of nursing that transcends the conventional way of thinking about the depth of nursing's contribution to society, the level of commitment and compassionate service to self and system and society.

When and if nursing and nurses reach this depth of being, beyond conventional knowing and doing; when and if nurses attain this new depth of wisdom; when we proceed with knowledge and practices that others do not know or see, we then have a responsibility to offer it to others, to interrupt the world's patterns of violence and noncaring. In this line of thinking, there is a connection between Caring (as connecting with, sustaining, and deepening our shared humanity) and Peace in the world.

In the Buddhist mind-set, nurses in this deeper model of "Being-the-work" become *bodhisattvas:* those who bless others and who become a blessing to self and others. These nurses then become Great Beings, heroines/heroes of an evolved *Caritas Consciousness* who are awake and actively affecting the entire universal field of humanity. This may seem far-fetched to many, but it is an emerging model of awakening and evolving within our caring humanity, away from our lethargy of nonawakened states. Thus, this level of awakening allows nursing to emerge into qualitative ontological states of wholeness. I share this view, in that my personal shift toward a deeper inner awakening leads me to introduce these notions so that others who study this work in depth can understand what is behind the theory of caring at the wisdom level, beyond conventional everyday thinking about nursing as "doing."

With this shift, I will also mention that this deeper model of *Caritas* and wisdom leads us to use a different language, along with different practices. For example, in this model we seek ways to avoid clinical language that labels and reduces humans and human experiences. The use of the formalized clinical language of nursing's past preoccupation has lost the capacity for beauty, grace, for dreams, inspiration, hope, imagination, creativity, artistry, for evoking the human spirit. The use of nonclinical language vibrates at a different level, at a higher frequency than clinical-technical, sterile words. Thus, we are stretched to consider new depths of meaning, new experiences and insights, new relationships with the experiences and the humans we encounter. Nonclinical language invites and takes us into words and worlds conventional languages cannot convey. Thus, we need words that are not "fixed," to avoid words that cannot convey higher vibrations of our humanity and the universality of our human spirit.

This view, this notion of "Being-the-Field" for caring-healing, is noble work for an ancient and noble profession in a new era in human history. However, it takes work and skills and depth of insight and wisdom to ponder and manifest. Once one enters into this thinking about and pondering such wisdom for nursing, we are in a new space for contributing to society and the world. In this model, we stop and pause in the midst of our most hurried and harried moments. We seek to bring calm and soothing, loving tones to the environmental field in the midst of crises, disease, pain, and suffering.

"It is returning, at last it is coming home to me—my own Self and those parts of it that have long been abroad and scattered among all things and accidents" (Nietzsche, *Thus Spoke Zarathustra*). However, it has to be acknowledged that to authentically engage in and sustain personal/professional practices guided by *Caritas Consciousness*, one needs skills. It is mandatory to cultivate personal practices so we are prepared to carry out the work in ways that are "biogenically" meaningful—that is, that are life giving and life receiving.

As part of the preparation for this practice of *Caritas*, I developed "touchstones" for setting our intentionality and consciousness for caring-healing. These touchstones were developed at the request of a hospital that was using my theory as a practice model for nursing and wanted to give the nurses something as a touchstone to prepare them for caring but also to remind them to continue to care. I developed the card shown as Table 4.1 for nurses, which is now more available to others. These sayings can be affirmations or can serve as a tool of sorts to begin to step more intentionally into the *Caritas* framework.

A preparatory practice such as the one set forth in Table 4.1 and the accompanying CD is only one way to enter into this kind of evolved awareness. It is only one entry into cultivating *Caritas Consciousness*. As we each step more fully into such affirmative practices of intentionality and evolving consciousness, we can expand and evolve into more formal experiences and practices.

BEGINNING CENTERING EXERCISE*

Another exercise that goes to a more focused level is the practice of "Centering." This exercise is another way to enter into and cultivate Loving-Kindness and Equanimity toward self and others. The exercise can also serve as both a starting point and a continuing guide for sustaining such caring-healing practices.

Since the universe is holographic, so is our role in it. In developing our own caring-healing practices and *Caritas Consciousness*, we are affecting the entire universe, from our own piece of personal and professional work, wherever we are; we are participating in and contributing to the universal field of infinity that surrounds us all. We need tools and skills to equip us to invoke and participate in becoming and holding the radiating field of loving-caring consciousness that affects the whole. Such cultivated preparatory work helps manifest *Caritas* energy of LOVE and compassion, elevating a higher/deeper awareness and presence, transcending fear and low-energy, ego-dominated controlling thoughts.

---

* The accompanying CD can serve as a guide to centering.

Table 4.1. Touchstones: Setting Intentionality and Consciousness for Caring and Healing

Caring in the Beginning

- Begin the day with silent gratitude; set your intentions to be open to give and receive all that you are here to give and receive this day; intend to bring your full self, in the day-to-day moments of this day; cultivating a loving, caring consciousness toward your self and all others who enter your path.

Caring in the Middle

- Take quiet moments to "center," to empty out, to be still with yourself before entering a patient's room or when entering a meeting; cultivate a loving-caring consciousness toward each person and each situation you encounter throughout the day; make an effort "to see" who the spirit-filled person is behind the patient/colleague.
- Return to these loving-centered intentions again and again, throughout the day, helping yourself to remember why you are here.
- In the middle of stressful moments, remember to breathe; ask for guidance when unsure, confused, and frightened; forgive and bless each situation.
- Let go of that which you cannot control.

Caring in the End

- At the end of the day, fold these intentions into your heart; commit yourself to cultivating a loving-caring practice for yourself.
- Use whatever has presented itself to you this day as lessons to teach you to grow more deeply into your own humanity and inner wisdom.
- At the end of the day, offer gratitude for all that has entered the sacred circle of your life and work this day.
- Bless, release, and dedicate the day to a higher, deeper order of the great sacred circle of life.

Caring Continuing

- Create your own intentions and your own authentic practices to prepare your *Caritas Consciousness;* find your individual spiritual path toward cultivating caring consciousness and meaningful experiences in your life and work and the world.

Source: Jean Watson © 2002.

CENTERING EXERCISE

A Centering exercise is one way to enter into, prepare for, and begin a more formal cultivation of the practice of Loving-Kindness and Equanimity as professional *Caritas Consciousness.*

To begin, you can either lie down or sit upright in a comfortable, alert position. Close your eyes and become aware of your body; fall into your body, softly allowing yourself to feel your body settled and grounded, knowing you are supported.

As you close your eyes to the outer world, open your inner eye and investigate what is happening in your inner mind-body self. To experience this, do a gentle body scan to be alert to your body position and let yourself breathe into all parts of your body, releasing tension, relaxing and settling and softening your body and your gentle awareness toward yourself and your body, offering loving, kind thoughts to self for this moment of stillness within and without.

As you continue to take deep but gentle breaths, on the out breath release everything in the outer world that you brought into this space, then release all the inner chatter. Just be still, breathing in and out, emptying out and filling up. As you breathe in, become gently aware that you are breathing in new life, new breath of life, spirit, energy of the universe. If you wish to have inner peace and to calm and relax any tension, you can do so on your out breath. By exhaling, we can obtain a state of restfulness even in the midst of inner and outer tension.

From this quiet place, gently continue to watch your breath, rising up and falling away. In gently and quietly attending to breath alone, one is connecting with the rhythm of the universe in that everything, everything, is rising up and falling away, just like the breath. In connecting with the natural rhythm of all of life, one is opening self to connection with the universe and the infinite wellspring of gratitude, loving-kindness, and equanimity.

As you continue to breathe, allow all thoughts, emotions, images that cross your awareness to rise up and fall away. In this quiet, still point, the in-between place, this void is where we access our deep source of creativity; it is where new awareness energy can manifest from spirit to material plane; it is where miracles occur, where we access the single point field and align with the universe.

We can access this space and awareness through this simple, brief, conscious, intentional, alert releasing practice of just stopping in the moment, quieting down, and breathing.

In connecting with breath, we breathe in spirit, the breath of life itself.

- Breathing alone can be a meditation.

- Breathing can be a mantra.

- Breathing is a miracle of life.

In breathing, we are both inhaling and exhaling; we are both empty and full. We are releasing that which has already passed, opening up vibratory space for new breath, new experience. Exhaling is a conscious letting go, surrendering to that which is; inhaling is opening to and connecting with the larger, deeper, complex pattern of life energy in infinite universe. It is this restful state that leads to a consciousness of equanimity—acquiring a mindfulness of noninterference with what is rising up and falling away in your inner and outer awareness; rather than cultivation, equanimity becomes a form of gentle acceptance of what is, a matter-of-factness without having to resist or avoid or alter what is. It is a form of surrendering to that which is in fact operating in our lives without trying to alter it, a form of radical permission to let things be, reminding me of the Beatles lyric "Let it be, let it be / Speaking words of wisdom, let it be."

In this place/space of letting it be, we become more fluid with our emotions and our body. We become alert and receptive; yet, like flowing water, we face life's vicissitudes; we prevent coagulating and setting our experiences, allowing them permission to pass, realizing everything is impermanent.

By the simple act of being still, connecting with that "still point" we all have deep inside, we open up to Source. In this simple act of gently watching the rising up and falling away of the breath, we empty out and realize deep inside how good it is to be still, to dwell in silence with the mystery and miracle of just breathing.

This simple, brief act alone, in the midst of our busy pace, can change our consciousness, preparing us to be present to whatever is in front of us to do/be; we are more able to witness our own self and shift our consciousness in a given moment when hurried, fearful, confused, conflicted, hurt, and so on. We can return again and again to this quiet, still point, allowing the feelings and the situation to be. Becoming watchful of the rising up and falling away of everything with alertness and presence, we are more able to respond appropriately to the presenting situation rather than reacting from a place of fear or anger or resentment.

In this experience, we discover that when we are able to cultivate this basic practice of Centering, things begin to change around us. So, as we change the way we are able to empty out, breathe, and release, we are more present in the moment. Then we affect the way we and others are able to be and to act. We are more able to alertly "read-the-field" in the midst of chaos, in the moment.

We can start a simple process and practice of Centering in the moment by a simple pause, *breathing,* and emptying out. We learn how to connect with, learn how to hold that still point, how to hold the void, that miracle point between the in breath and the out breath. It is in this space, this void, this still point, this empty space, where something new can happen in the moment (rather than a closing down or setting, congealing, and freezing of self and situation).

Finally, when you are ready, come back into your present space, feeling more open, more gentle, more alert, more peaceful, more present, more conscious and intentional about your *Caritas* Being.

Within the practice of *Caritas Nursing,* which embraces such meditative practices of equanimity and loving-kindness toward self and other, we have advantages in our daily life. Our mindful, caring presence affects others; it increases our level of energy and creativity for our work without wasting or dribbling away our life energy–life force; it helps us observe the work with more clarity and discernment without reacting inappropriately. It helps us to "Be Present."

One of the first requirements for stepping into a model of caring-healing and *Caritas Consciousness* is to be fully present in the moment, more open and available to self and situation. This simple exercise, done as a formal practice or as an instant connection to stop and breathe and let go, is foundational to authentic presence required for professional practice.

ADDITIONAL EXERCISE: CULTIVATION OF
A PRACTICE OF GRATITUDE AND FORGIVENESS

Another exercise, an extension of the previous basic centering experience, can lead to deeper growth in one's authentic practice and preparation for *Caritas Consciousness*: the Practice of Gratitude, Surrender, and Forgiveness. We can extend this same exercise to cultivation of a sense of gratitude and forgiveness of all, opening again to breathing, quieting down, and connecting with the infinite Source and that still point inside, the space between the in breath and the out breath.

As you continue to breathe, become once again gently aware of the impermanence of everything, the expanding and contracting of the breath, connecting with the rhythm of the universe. Rising up and falling away.

In this quiet place, from this still point deep inside, just appreciate yourself: all of your hard work, your efforts, dreams, challenges, hopes, frustrations, failures, disappointments, losses, and suffering— all of it. Just appreciate what all has brought you to this moment in time. Just appreciate yourself and who you are.

From this quiet place, ask yourself if there is any situation, thing, or person, including yourself, you need to forgive; then do it now, in the quiet space within—allowing yourself to forgive, bless, surrender, and release it to the universe so you are free of the hurt and pain of holding those feelings.

Continue to breathe.

Then, with your mind's eye, allow yourself to send out loving gratitude and forgiveness to others: family, other loved ones, colleagues, patients, any others in your field of awareness who need love and forgiveness—shower them with loving blessings.

Offer gratitude for all that is, all of your life and your lessons and blessings, feeling a sense of deep trust and inner peace from within that quiet place inside. Then, when you feel a sense of completion and when you are ready, send loving energy and kindness to all humans and all of life—from this deeper place of forgiveness, gratitude, surrender, and love. Radiate your inner peace and *Caritas Consciousness* to all those in your field and to the broader universe. Finally, when you are ready, return to this space more open, present, alert, and centered to continue what is in front of you to do.

These exercises serve as both a practice guide and an invitation to cultivate and prepare self for the deep nature of authentic caring and healing that is fueled by a deep, abiding love of self and other and all of life. These exercises can be a starting point for the more formal practice of Mindfulness–Insight Meditation: Loving-Kindness and Equanimity.

TOWARD A FORMAL PRACTICE OF MINDFULNESS–INSIGHT MEDITATION: LOVING-KINDNESS AND EQUANIMITY*

You can search the whole universe and not find a single being more worthy of love than yourself.

THE BUDDHA (QUOTED IN KORNFIELD 2002:101)

If one wanted to explore formal meditation as a lifelong preparatory practice for sustaining and expanding one's *Caritas Consciousness* for self and other, one formal practice with which I am acquainted is *Vipassana: Mindfulness and Insight Meditation.*

Without getting technical, this form of meditation is known as Vipassana Meditation, which is derived from one of the schools of Buddhism; however, it is not tied to a religion per se. It has followers from around the world, from all walks of life, from all religions and even those with no religion. It is increasingly being discovered for personal, professional, and clinical applications of self-awareness, evolution of consciousness, and mindfulness in action, as well as for specific clinical conditions—for example, chronic and acute pain management, addiction, compulsions, depression, and related areas.

This form of meditation is recommended not only because I have experienced it and continue to practice it but because it is directly relevant to professionals preparing themselves to be present and mindful in caring-healing work. It is closely related to learning to live the Theory to Be/Become the *Caritas Consciousness* we wish to be.

Therefore, it is important to find ways to cultivate a consciousness of *Caritas*: loving-kindness and equanimity if one is to authentically practice within this paradigm. That is not to say that this is the only form of preparation. There are unlimited approaches to prepare self, but mindfulness meditation is one timeless approach that has lasting

---

* This section was influenced by personal experiences, tapes, books, and the Web site of Shinzen Young, my formal teacher, at http://Shinzen.org.

and profound experiences for the practitioner and his or her work in the world. Thus, this practice leads to transformation of self at a deep level; transformation of practitioners is necessary before the systems can be transformed.

Equanimity

Some are unfamiliar with the word "equanimity." It is derived from a Latin word and refers to an inner state of balance, an internal sense of balanced spirit. It is a process of noninterference with what IS. There is no freezing or fixing or congealing of the awareness, just observing and letting it be, allowing self to be in harmony with the natural flow of a subjective state (Young personal communication, 2006).

Equanimity with Unpleasant Sensations

When one is able (through meditative-mindfulness practices) to intentionally create equanimity in body or mind toward its subjective sensations, allowing whatever is there to be observed without interference, then there is natural flow of the process. For example, if there is pain or discomfort, worry or fear, the sensations flow more easily as you observe them without interference, without judging them. It is almost as if you have mercy toward both them and yourself. In this process, you begin to understand more than intellectually that all sensations are energetically expanding and contracting, but you actually experience the flow and movement. When one is distressed or suffering, the practice of equanimity lessens the suffering, decreasing the discomfort in body or mind.

Equanimity with Pleasant Sensations

Likewise, when you apply equanimity to pleasant sensations without interfering, they too flow more readily and easily and offer deeper fulfillment. Together, then, equanimity works to both lessen suffering and increase pleasure by the simple practice of mindfulness, applying loving-kindness to self and the process.

Without the practice of Equanimity, one cannot fully access the intrinsic wellspring of loving-kindness for *Caritas Consciousness*.

As one allows the sensations to flow, that flow forms a kind of psychic purification of the feelings so one is more authentically available to experience loving-kindness as the wellspring that helps to access the inside rather than a superficial external facade.

It does not work to "put on" an overcoat of loving-kindness when anger, hurt, despair, worry, and similar feelings are present. Only after those feelings have been allowed to flow can the deep wellspring of authentic *Caritas* emerge, radiating out from self to others and one's field (Young personal communication, 2006).

LOVING-KINDNESS

Loving-kindness gives birth to a natural compassion. The compassionate heart holds the pain and sorrow of our life and of all beings with mercy and tenderness. . . . It is the tender heart that has the power to transform the world.

KORNFIELD (2002:102)

Considering the first *Caritas Process* in depth and accessing the intent related to loving-kindness and equanimity invite a form of mindfulness/meditation in action. Exploring this aspect of meditation for *Caritas Consciousness* is one way to attend to this foundational way of *Being* as the basis for caring, healing, and wholeness. It is a core practice and process that prepares us with the skill and ability to commit to and engage in lifelong compassionate human service that is life giving and life receiving.

Everyone has an intrinsic wellspring of loving-kindness, caring, and friendliness. However, this basic intrinsic way of Being often gets coated over and buried under conventional social customs and workplace norms. At the same time, loving-kindness is a natural state of being and living, in that when we feel it fully, it brings joy and peace to our lives and to those around us. The challenge within a caring-healing professional practice and a special challenge for a *Caritas Consciousness* model is learning how to access these feelings directly so you are radiating that energy to self and to the field around you.

Remember the truism: the universe is a hologram. Then, the holographic notion applies here: if the part is in the whole and vice versa, if even one practitioner prepares self for *Caritas Consciousness* as the basis for professional caring practices, that one nurse is helping transform and affect the entire field. Imagine what it would be like if nurses collectively engaged in meditative practices to cultivate *Caritas Consciousness.*

First at the personal level, then at the unit level, then across units, spreading throughout the entire system, then across systems, across settings in various parts of the world.

Nurses with informed *Caritas Consciousness* could literally transform entire systems, contributing to worldwide changes through their own practices of Being, thus "seeing" and *doing* things differently—holding a different consciousness, radiating different messages, affecting the subtle energetic environment, spreading healing, wholeness, forgiveness, beauty, love, kindness, equanimity. In this awareness, this awakening, nurses are literally *Becoming the Caritas field.*

Once one has experienced such a cultivated sense of loving-kindness, one's heart of compassion is open and bubbles over into one's life circumstances. However, as mentioned before, one cannot artificially invoke loving thoughts if one is in pain, angry, sad, despairing or fearful, worrisome, and so on. One cannot paint over a veneer of hurts; rather, he or she must allow pain to emerge, whereby it is both released and absorbed into the vibrating space of energy flow.

That is the purpose of mindfulness meditation: to learn to use this practice when in a negative space, to find ways to access feelings and subjective sensations without dwelling there, without setting, masking, coating over, or freezing those sensations. The congealing of sensations and fighting off, ignoring, or avoiding feelings create more suffering. The meditation practices proposed here help one access and observe all sensations, discovering their vibratory, energetic nature rising up and falling away; either by visualizing these movements or literally experiencing the sensations, we transform the emotional experience.

Once one connects with and practices noninterference (equanimity), the energy and feelings move through a sense of completion and closure that is a form of sweet release; these sensations can be both observed and felt. Then, empty vibratory space opens up internally, allowing one to authentically access and feel the loving-kindness and equanimity one longs to feel, which flow naturally once the negative space has been emptied out.

Once the other feelings have finished welling up and passing away, loving-kindness feelings pour into the vibrating space where before one held pain. Once this practice has been cultivated, one is able to relate to others with this practice as a professional *Caritas* act.

As we learn to cultivate the practice of Loving-Kindness and Equanimity as part of our preparation for *Caritas Consciousness*, we have entered a new level of personal and professional transformation that affects everything we know, do, and "be" in our work and world. Strategies for formal meditation practices are available through a variety of workshops, books, and tapes and on the Internet.

I especially recommend the Web site of Shinzen Young (http://shinzen.org). He has audiotapes online; his core practices, which one can experience by listening to him, are available at no cost; there are also written materials and information about Vipassana Meditation, Mindfulness Meditation, equanimity, and so on. His many other books, tapes, and similar materials can also be ordered on the site.

The first *Caritas Process*: Cultivation of Loving-Kindness and Equanimity, has introduced simple beginning touchstones, exercises, affirmations, Centering exercises, and an overview of Mindfulness Meditation. Options exist to step into this personal/professional preparation at whatever level, whenever one is ready. To pursue this practice systematically and formally is a lifelong journey. A formal commitment to find one's own practice and preparation for this work can make all the difference in one's career. Meditation is an invitation for lifelong personal growth so we become the living theory of caring, the ones accessing the *Caritas Field/Becoming the Caritas Field* in our work and our world.

CHAPTER FIVE

From **CARATIVE FACTOR 2:** *Installation of Faith and Hope*
to **CARITAS PROCESS 2:** *Being Authentically Present:*
Enabling, Sustaining, and Honoring the Faith, Hope, and Deep
Belief System and the Inner-Subjective Life World of Self/Other

---

Hope springs eternal not because of the nature of the world, but
because of the nature of God. . . . [T]he light of Creation does
not emanate from the material world, and so it is useless to seek it
there.

MARIANNE WILLIAMSON

If you lose hope, somehow you lose the vitality that keeps life
moving; you lose that courage to be, that quality that helps you to
go on in spite of all.

MARTIN LUTHER KING JR.

Hope is the thing with feathers
That perches in the Soul.
And sings the tune without the words,
And never stops at all.

EMILY DICKINSON

The original Carative Factor of faith and hope is closely tied to the expanded language that seeks to make it a little more explicit with respect to the level of authenticity required for human presence in the midst of the need for faith and hope, making more explicit the importance of honoring the deep belief system and subjective inner-life world of meaning the other person holds for his or her life and purpose and the presenting situation in which that person happens to find him- or herself. Another's situation could be any of our situations, eliciting compassion and deep understanding and reaching out to other, honoring his or her belief in the right outcome for self. This *Caritas Process* likewise honors the belief system of the nurse, inviting the practitioner to connect with that which sustains him or her when in need of faith and hope to draw upon. All of us need faith and hope to carry us through the vicissitudes and slings and arrows of the human earth-plane existence.

This expanded *Caritas Process* is closely related to the foundational humanistic-altruistic value system and to loving-kindness and equanimity as consciousness. These are the touchstones, the foundation and core processes that carry us into and through the work of human caring-healing and life experiences of birthing, living, being, dying.

We cannot ignore the importance of hope and faith and the role they play in people's lives, especially when faced with the unknowns, mysteries, and crises of illness, pain, loss, stress, despair, grief, trauma, death, and so on. That is why this value concept is included as core to a professional model of nursing and to Caring Science: *Caritas Consciousness*.

One of the ways we feel hope is to offer hope to another. Often we discover that in this moment, because we are here we are the hope; we may become the hope for someone who is isolated, alone, abandoned in the prison of his or her despair and illness, fear and suffering. By being sensitive to our own presence and *Caritas Consciousness,* not only are we able to offer and enable another to access his or her own belief system of faith-hope for the person's healing, but we may be the one who makes the difference between hope and despair in a given moment.

As noted in the original text (Watson 1979), the therapeutic (healing) effects of faith-hope have been documented throughout history. Hippocrates thought an ill person's mind and soul should be inspired before the illness was treated. Aristotle was aware that the theater had a therapeutic effect on a person who became involved with performance and drama. Asclepius, the Greek god of medicine, was often pictured with his two daughters—Hygeia, the goddess of health, and Panacea, the goddess of healing. Hygeia guarded health through self-discipline and a good environment; Panacea used drugs and manipulations to heal (Ackerknecht 1968:xvii). *Panacea* has continuing meanings associated with cures for ills and difficulties; the panacea effect is commonly referred to when one cannot explain the direct cause of cures and improvement in a patient's health.

In ancient Egypt, the priest and the physician were the same person. For many centuries Egyptian medicine was closely associated with religion and faith.

Faith and hope have traditionally been important in treatment to relieve the symptoms of illness; medicine itself was secondary to magic, incantations, spells, and prayers. Miracles of faith appear often in the Bible, as well as in more recent times. The role of prayer has taken on both scientific and spiritual meaning, offering hope and faith to millions around the world every day in many life situations.

New explanations of and research on prayer, distant healing, and related phenomena of faith and hope, previously unexplained in conventional medicine, are taking on new dimensions through the work of Larry Dossey and others in the medical and religious communities (Dossey 1993). Other related studies are increasingly being replicated, making a strong case for the role of healing words and belief in prayer, locally or at a distance. This work on prayer and healing words is consistent with ancient and even modern practices of treatment through suggestion, power of thoughts, visualization, imagery, and belief that transcends time and science.

Other ancient approaches to treatment and cures, such as the Babylonians' astrological approach, were also based on supernatural explanations of the causes of and cures for disease and illness. We still see evidence of soul retrieval, chants, and other devices used to call off evil spirits, as well as diverse efforts to bring forth or call out help from the nonphysical spirit world to the physical plane, to reestablish harmony and balance and healing.

Mesmer, in the late eighteenth century, was the first to publicly draw attention to the importance of mental treatments as having a direct bearing on illness. He was considered the father of hypnosis and came to treat illness, after trying several different approaches, through what was and is still known as "mesmerism," or suggestion—later explored as the phenomenon still known clinically as hypnosis. Hypnosis continues to be used and researched today for addressing a variety of medical and psychological conditions—for example, the relief of minor headache pain, the elimination of major symptoms of illness, and use as an anesthetic during surgical procedures. The effects of hypnosis and placebos, both forms of suggestion, are linked to authentic presence and enabling faith and hope.

More recently, numerous studies have shown the role and power of (caring) relationships in affecting the outcome of illness and diagnosis. Caring relationships (Carative Factor 4) explore the importance of relationship but within the context of faith-hope. The presence of a caring professional may be a source of enabling, sustaining, and honoring the other's belief system and source of hope.

Many believe that when all else fails, something "still needs to be done." In many instances that something is having faith in a person, a health regime, or a belief system to carry them through.

Some have posited that the present era is the "beginning of the end of physical (Era I) medicine" (where the focus is on the body as machine and on physical-material, external medical interventions), as we have known it to be over the past century. We must increasingly acknowledge worldwide that allopathic medicine, as practiced in the Westernized, scientific world, is only one of a number of ways people seek treatment and cures. Millions of people continue to believe that the movement of the stars and constellations, if properly interpreted (astrological predictions), can reveal their fate. Intelligent people have sought nonscientific approaches when faced with unknowns and life crises, especially when the condition seems hopeless and nothing more can be done "medically." However, people can always call upon their source of hope from their belief system. It seems as though when people are ill or threatened or in crisis, they "go home" culturally and internally, subjectively resorting to their inner deep belief system, regardless of whether it is "rational" or "irrational."

Today, conventional Western medicine is using multiple modalities as adjuncts to other scientific approaches or, at best, in conjunction with allopathic practices. The growing field now commonly referred to as Integrated Medicine, or mind-body-spirit medicine, is using such holistic modalities as meditation, energy medicine, acupuncture, Reiki treatments, biofeedback, homeopathy, diet, exercise, visualization, intentional consciousness, touch–noncontact touch, relationship therapy, and numerous other procedures and practices. Belief remains at the heart of all practices. These approaches build upon, but also extend and transcend, conventional allopathic medicine and at some level draw upon and reinforce the deep belief system of the one being cared for.

Many of these so-called holistic modalities are grounded in a different worldview than the Western belief system; they incorporate spiritual-religious dimensions and other supernatural unknowns, thus contributing all the more to the complexities and importance of honoring deep beliefs, perceptions, and subjective meanings. Many of these practices are ancient and pre-modern but have been rediscovered as contributing to healing and wholeness and broad health outcomes. Whether from ancient Greek and Chinese medicine or modern nursing founded by Nightingale, they are based on the wisdom that the body has the power at some deep intrinsic level to heal itself. This belief is often what people return to in calling upon their hope and faith, their belief in miracles as a source of strength.

In *Caritas Consciousness*, the nurse honors and seeks to discover what is meaningful and important for a particular person. The person's beliefs are never discarded or dismissed as insignificant in the treatment and caring process. Indeed, they are encouraged, respected, and enabled as significant in promoting healing and wholeness regardless of medical diagnosis, situation, and cure outcomes.

The nurse practicing within a Caring Science context knows that the healing power of belief and hope can never be overlooked but

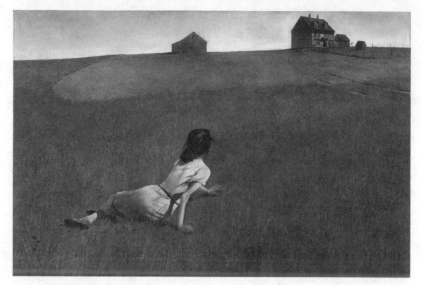

Figure 7. Christina's World, *by Andrew Wyeth. Collection, The Museum of Modern Art, New York City.*

must be incorporated into the caring relationship and caring practices. Reinforcing faith-hope and honoring the deep belief system of self and other build upon and draw from the humanistic altruism and *Caritas Consciousness* of *Caritas Process* 1: Practice of loving-kindness and equanimity to promote professional, ethical caring. These factors and processes complement each other and further contribute to the third Carative Factor/*Caritas Process,* related to the sensitivity and spiritual growth of the practitioner.

CHAPTER SIX

From **CARATIVE FACTOR 3:** *Cultivation of*
Sensitivity to Oneself and Others
to **CARITAS PROCESS 3:** *Cultivation of One's*
Own Spiritual Practices and Transpersonal
Self, Going Beyond Ego-Self

This factor/process is a lifelong journey and a big order for professional practice. Here I continue to teach what I continually need to learn. This journey is a process of evolving and honoring one's own inner needs, listening to the still, small voice inside, connecting with our deepest source for awakening into our *Being* and *Becoming*. In this *Caritas Process* (CP) we return to the first CP: cultivation of loving-kindness and equanimity and entering into practices to cultivate them. In doing so, CP 3 naturally leads to a spiritual practice and becomes transpersonal; such a process connects us with spirit and Source and that which is greater than ego.

However, without attending to and cultivating one's own spiritual growth, insight, mindfulness, and spiritual dimension of life, it is very difficult to be sensitive to self and other. Without this lifelong process and journey, we can become hardened and brittle and can close down our compassion and caring for self and other.

Thus, this *Caritas Process* seeks to make explicit that our professional commitment to caring-healing and the wholeness of Being/doing/knowing cannot be complete or mature without focusing on this evolving aspect of our personal and professional growth.

INTEGRATION OF FACTORS AND PROCESSES

To be human is to feel. All too often we allow ourselves to *think our thoughts but not feel our feelings.* The primary way to develop sensitivity and a need for spiritual practices is to pay attention to our feelings and thoughts—painful as well as happy ones. We need to recognize the mental images we hold in our minds and our consciousness and carry with us; we need to be more mindful of internal scripts—what do we say to our self? What is the nature of the internal chatter?

As we adopt some spiritual practice to connect with the inner self and inner life world, we open to that which goes beyond the outer-worldly physical dimension. We then seek a higher/deeper source for inner wisdom and our own truths.

Many people do not fulfill their potential. They tend to look for solutions outside themselves. But the source of maturity, wisdom, reflection, insight, and mindfulness for developing an evolved consciousness is within. To begin is to look within, to not be afraid of the shadow-and-light side of our humanity; what makes us more deeply human and humane is to make contact with, honor, and offer loving-kindness to self, even those aspects we fear or do not like. Without attending to this aspect of caring and *Caritas Consciousness* there is no growth, and we will have limited success in working with the humanity of others if we cannot accept and love self first.

This process of ongoing spiritual development is the foundation for caring, compassion, and transpersonal human-to-human connections with another. This dimension and process help us to "see" who the spirit-filled person is beyond the outer physical elements, beyond the patient, diagnosis, and so on. One must be able to connect with, see, and accept that all feelings and thoughts are continually rising up and falling away. However, through this practice and process we can experience the reality that we have feelings and thoughts, but they do not define who we are. We have thoughts; we have feelings; we have a body; but we are more than our thoughts, our feelings, and our body. We are embodied spirit. Or, as Teilhard de Chardin reminded us, we are spiritual beings having an earthly experience.

If a nurse is not sensitive to her or his own feelings, it is difficult to be sensitive to another. It is when we are unaware, unreflective about self and life, that we harden our self to the feelings of others and close down our hearts, making us insensitive and even cruel—just when others may be most in need of our loving-kindness, concern, compassion, and sensitivity. When this occurs the nurse often forms detached professional relationships, camouflaging potential conflicts and even contributing to a toxic situation or an unhealthy work environment.

While the Carative Factor of sensitivity is core, it is enhanced and serves as the foundation for spiritual growth, maturity, and reflective and mindful practices when expanded to *Caritas Consciousness*; thus, this third *Caritas Process* extends the third factor's meaning and focus. This process and factor cannot be taken for granted, so they need to be identified as the core of professional human-to-human relationships and caring-healing practices. All of these factors and evolved processes overlap and are holographic in nature, in that each one resides within the whole of the other and the whole of the Caring Science paradigm resides within each of the factors/processes.

EDUCATIONAL NOTE/REMINDER

In many ways, the third, fourth, and fifth Carative Factors, re-revised and reframed as *Caritas Processes,* can be combined. They are all part of a holographic whole; they are all mutually interdependent. They each, in their own way, speak to human ontological relational aspects of the nurse's development of self to be in *Caritas Consciousness*, to practice *Caritas Nursing*. All of these dimensions are necessary to enact a living philosophy, theory, and ethic that seek to sustain professional caring-healing in relation with self and other. For intellectual-conceptual organizational purposes, however, I have identified them as separate factors/processes in that I think, in their own way, each merits attention and discussion. However, they all are interactive and

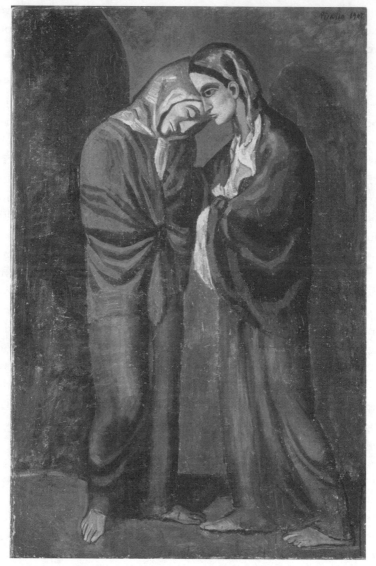

Figure 8. The Meeting, *by Pablo Picasso (1881–1973).* © *ARS, NY. Location, Hermitage, St. Petersburg, Russia. Photo credit, Scala/Art Resource, New York.*

simultaneously holographic. Thus, we enter into discussion of the fourth Carative Factor, now extending to *Caritas Process* 4, which intersects directly with all the others that have come before.

CHAPTER SEVEN

From **CARATIVE FACTOR 4:** *Developing a Helping-Trusting Relationship*
to **CARITAS PROCESS 4:** *Developing and Sustaining a Helping-Trusting Caring Relationship*

A person becomes a person in the encounter with other persons and in no other way.

SOURCE UNKNOWN

The central task of health professions education—in nursing, medicine, dentistry, public health, psychology, social work, and the allied health professions—must be to help students, faculty, and practitioners learn how to form caring, healing relationships with patients, their communities and with each other, and with themselves . . . the knowledge, skills, and values necessary for effective relationships. . . . Developing practitioners, able to mature as reflective learners and professionals who understand the patient as a person . . . [also] understand the essential nature of healing relationships.

PEW FETZER REPORT (1994:39)

Relationship-centered caring is considered intrinsic to healing and the foundation for a deeper level of health care reform that goes beyond the superficial economic focus of change. The focus on relationship includes multiple layers of relationship:

- Practitioner to self
- Practitioner to patient
- Practitioner to community
- Practitioner to practitioner.

The need exists to develop and sustain caring relationships as the core of professional practices in all health professions (Pew Fetzer Report 1994). In modifying the language of this Carative Factor, the main changes are related to making more explicit the authentic caring aspect of the helping-trusting relationship.

In conventional psycho-therapeutic processes and protocols, it is possible to learn techniques of communication, how to succeed in having someone disclose his or her feelings, and so forth. However, in *Caritas Consciousness*, authenticity and genuineness of human connection and responses are necessary as an ethic; the authenticity of self reveals the integrity of the professional. This is an ingredient for a caring moment and opens up transpersonal dimensions of caring-healing.

Transpersonal caring moments can be existential turning points; these moments are reverential in honoring the unity of the whole person: mind-body-spirit. Thus, this dimension may be extremely critical, but it can also be threatening to practitioners if they are not practicing within *Caritas Consciousness* and if the *Caritas Processes* or Carative Factors are not cultivated. Developing a caring relationship requires skill and ontological human caring competencies; it is not about technique per se.

Rather, authentic caring relationship building is concerned with deepening our humanity; it is about processes of being-becoming more humane, compassionate, aware, and awake to our own and others' human dilemma. It is about human presence, authentic listening and hearing, being present for another in the moment. It is about "reading the field." It is about being reflective, mindful, and skillful mid-step, mid-sentence, mid-action when connecting with another person. Such competencies and skill in connecting with another generate trust and safety. It is a life-giving, life-receiving, human-to-human, spirit-to-spirit connection that goes beyond the physical-ego level. These skills and this consciousness for relationship involve ontological competencies, as presented earlier. Such relationship building is about first understanding self as a critical variable in any care situation. How to translate one's own self-awareness, sensitivity, and loving-consciousness into informed moral practice in relation to self and other is a major task of professional practice.

This process, this consciousness, this skill of being-in-relation is fundamental and essential to any caring-healing relationship, as it is often *the* relationship itself that is healing rather than the external interventions alone. A body of empirical evidence supports what many have ethically, intuitively, and experientially known for centuries—that the *quality* of the relationship with another person is one of the most significant elements in determining helping effectiveness. At the least, the research indicates that relationship is a strong predictor of outcome, beyond the actual therapy; thus, at the very least, interventions interact with the relationship for the most therapeutic, healing outcomes (Herman 1993; Horvath and Symonds 1991; Luborsky et al. 1986; Martin, Garske, and Davis 2000; Orlinsky and Howard 1985; Strupp and Hadley 1979).

In this sense, the caring relationship can be considered an intervention in and of itself, or at least a core ingredient. For example, some research in the medical literature has indicated that "better health," functional behavior, and subjective evaluations are related to physician-patient communication (Kaplan, Greenfield, and Ware 1989, cited in Quinn et al. 2003). The nursing literature has a great deal of information and publications related to relationship and caring, even though few are controlled studies. In general, the Caring Science literature in the field is closely aligned and consistent with renewed scientific and educational interest in caring relationships and healing outcomes (Pew Fetzer Report 1994; Samueli Conference on Definitions and Standards in Healing Research 2002).

The Carative Factors/*Caritas Processes* discussed earlier, such as mindfulness, loving-kindness, sensitivity, hope, and faith, all contribute to the quality of an authentic caring relationship. Nevertheless, the relationship itself merits study and attention. Whether we see nursing as the Philosophy and Science of Caring or caring as the Philosophy and Science of Nursing, either way we are required to consider seriously the empirical as well as the ethical, theoretical, and experiential evidence related to development of an authentic caring-healing relationship.

Of the many problems that can arise in nursing, perhaps one of the most common is the failure to establish rapport, being insensitive, unable to connect or create an alliance with another. Put another way, a major problem is the lack of a reflective, mindful awareness of how one's presence and consciousness toward self and other can and do affect the nature and outcome of one's relationship with another, whether the other is a colleague, a patient, or a family member. It is common knowledge, as well as empirical knowledge, that a patient who feels the nurse *truly, authentically* cares about and for the patient and sees who she or he is behind the patient status is more likely to establish trust, faith, and hope and sustain a caring relationship with the nurse. When one is able to engage in presence and truly listen to and hear another person's story, that may be the greatest healing gift of all. It is then that the other is far more likely to talk about sensitive matters—what is really bothering him or her behind the superficial words or overt behavior.

As the discipline of nursing has evolved to honor and develop the art and science of human caring, relationship itself has become core to professional practices. Indeed, the philosophical, theoretical, and scientific nursing literature now subsumes many constructs tied to healing: empathy, compassion, commitments, communication, humanistic-altruistic values, instilling faith and hope, sensitivity to self and other, respect, trust, love, patient- and person-centered relationships, and so on (Quinn et al. 2003).

Some of the more formal research on caring and outcomes was conducted by Swanson (1999), who described outcomes of caring and noncaring relationships. The meta-analysis showed that for patients who experienced caring, outcomes included:

- Emotional and spiritual well-being (dignity, self-control, personhood)
- Enhanced healing and enhanced relationship with others.

The consequences of noncaring were reported to be:

- Feelings of humiliation, fear
- Feeling out of control, desperate
- Feeling helpless, alienated, and vulnerable.

These same outcomes of caring and noncaring were mirrored by nurses. For example, for nurses practicing caring, the outcomes were:

- A sense of personal and professional satisfaction and fulfillment
- A love of nursing
- The ability to live out their own philosophy.

Consequences of noncaring for nurses were:

- Feeling hardened, oblivious, depressed
- Feeling frightened, brittle
- Feeling worn down. (Swanson 1999)

These findings continue to both haunt and remind us that effects of caring and relationship are critical to outcomes for patients and nurses alike. However, while a wealth of empirical, qualitative, theoretical, and philosophical data suggest the importance of the caring relationship to the health and well-being of nurses and their patients, it must be acknowledged that limited quantitative research supports these qualitative views and studies (Quinn et al. 2003). This situation is all the more an indicator for additional research within the Caring Science framework.

Such acknowledgment underscores the position that at a basic disciplinary level, the caring relationship is core to the meta-narrative that defines the ethics, values, and theoretical and philosophical norms for the profession. The fact that almost every extant nursing theory, professional nursing curriculum, and professional practice model emphasizes the caring relationship in some form, and the fact that qualitative studies continue to find the importance of that relationship, indicate that a core value, ethic, and essential behavior guide nursing's covenant and commitment to the public. While research of a quantitative nature continues to be needed, the lack of quantitative studies should not undermine the ethical, philosophical value commitment to sustain an authentic trusting-caring relationship with another; the caring relationship is foundational to any professional practice. Without attending to this core *Caritas Process*, nursing would cease to be a profession.

CHAPTER EIGHT

Theoretical Framework for Caritas/*Caring Relationship*

CARITAS / CARING RELATIONSHIP

Several conceptual and theoretical nursing/health-science frameworks in caring link caring and relationship with healing and broad health outcomes. The Caring Science context of my work has provided a foundation for research, practice, education, and nursing administration since the original text in 1979. This work has continued to evolve.

Within the context of a caring-healing relationship, the Caring Science model posits an energetic nature for *Caritas Consciousness*: that caring consciousness emanates an energy that radiates from one party to the other. It alters the field in the moment, helping patients access their inner healing potential. This healing potential is a natural process that has to do with "being-in-right-relation" (Quinn 1989). The caring relationship in this context preserves human dignity, wholeness, and integrity; it is characterized by the nurse's mindful, intentional presence and choice, in that the nurse can choose how to be in a caring moment. That decision can affect the relationship, for better or for worse. The transpersonal nature of the caring relationship occurs when the nurse is able to connect with the spirit of the other, that which is behind the patient, thus opening to a spirit-to-spirit connection that goes beyond the moment and becomes part of the universal, complex pattern of both their lives. The nurse and the patient carry those moments into their future, which informs their next experiences, perceptions, and so forth. Thus, both the nurse and the patient are changed as a result of the relationship and the nature of the experience (Watson 1985).

The transpersonal nature of the experience is connected with the nurse's ability to be authentically present in a way that reaches out to the other, transcending ego. This is the source of compassion, when one is able to connect transpersonally. The concepts of transpersonal and compassion are captured by Jack Kornfield: "Compassion arises naturally as 'quivering of the heart' in the face of pain, ours and another's. True compassion is not limited by the separateness of pity, nor by the fear of being overwhelmed. When we come to rest in the great heart of compassion, we discover a capacity to bear witness to, suffer with, and hold dear with our own vulnerable heart the sorrow and beauties of the world" (2002:103).

TRANSPERSONAL CARING RELATIONSHIP*

This section develops the theoretical views on the Transpersonal Caring Relationship, consistent with the emphasis on *Caritas Consciousness* as part of the fourth *Caritas Process* (CP), while making connections with other extant nursing theory.

Other contemporary nursing theories provide a view consistent with transpersonal, *Caritas*/Caring Consciousness notions discussed here. Newman and colleagues (1991) posited a unitary, transformative paradigm to contain nursing practice and research. In such a paradigm a phenomenon is viewed as a unitary, self-organizing field embedded in a larger, self-organizing field. Knowledge is personal and involves

---

* Parts of this section are extracted from Watson 2004a.

pattern recognition. It includes perceptions and what I would call the "phenomenal field"—the subjective and intersubjective meanings of both participants. Thus, any phenomenon has to be viewed as a whole, not as an additive sum of the parts to make a whole. These notions of interconnection, as well as holographic unitary views of the universe, are consistent with the theoretical dimensions of a transpersonal caring relationship. Newman's views of "health as expanding consciousness" and Martha Rogers's Unitary Science (Rogers 1970, 1994) are consistent with *Caritas Consciousness* in that caring and love call upon higher levels of consciousness for professional nursing and make connections between caring and healing/health/wholeness outcomes, transcending conventional outcomes of curing alone.

A transpersonal caring relationship is guided by an evolving *Caritas Consciousness*. It conveys a concern for the inner life world and subjective meaning of another; that other is fully embodied, that is, embodied spirit. The notion of transpersonal invites full loving-kindness and equanimity of one's presence-in-the-moment, with an understanding that a significant caring moment can be a turning point in one's life. It affects both nurse and patient and radiates out beyond the moment, connecting with the universal field of infinity to which we all belong and in which we dwell. Thus, the moment lives on.

Such an authentic spirit-to-spirit connection in a given moment transcends the personal ego level of professional control and opens the nurse's intelligent heart and head to what is really emerging and presenting itself in the now-moment. The transpersonal *Caritas Consciousness* nurse is more open, responsive, and sensitive to what is occurring—more able to "read the field," to pick up on subtleties in the field, to use all resources and draw upon all ways of knowing: empirical-technical, ethical, intuitive, personal, aesthetic, even spiritual knowing.

She or he is more able to enter into and stay within the other person's frame of reference; to shift from the functional, often routine, set procedure, agenda, or task and "see" and "hear" verbal and nonverbal cues; to attend to what is most important for the person behind the patient and the procedure. The nurse is alert and responsive to what is present and emerging for the other in this given-now-moment.

This shift of awareness and the ability to be present-in-the-now, in *this* moment, do not preclude the nurse from performing necessary tasks or procedures. Rather, transpersonal *Caritas Consciousness* actually expands the caring; indeed, in some, if not many, instances, transpersonal *Caritas Consciousness*, this acquired skill of *being present-in-the-now*, reduces the demands for caring. The care that is offered becomes more accurate, more focused, more appropriate, and generally more fulfilling for both nurse and patient. It can be healing, life giving, and life receiving.

Transpersonal *Caritas Consciousness* and relationship call for an authenticity of *Being and Becoming*—more fully human and humane, more openhearted, compassionate, sensitive, present, capable; more competent as a human; more able to dwell in silence, to engage in informed moral actions with pain, discomfort, emotional struggles, and suffering without turning away. These competencies, this consciousness, are related to the other Carative Factors and *Caritas Processes* and exist at the ethical, moral ontological level and demand for professional nursing caring practice. This consciousness offers a common search for meaning for healing, for relationships of all kinds, for illness, pain, suffering, loss, death, vulnerability, and so forth.

The common ineffable human experiences we all share are those human tasks related to how to live and how to face death and dying, whether our own struggles for living and dying or those of a stranger, a patient, or a loved one. These are the *Caritas* quests for the deep reality we face in the nursing profession. Often, these are the unstated, underdeveloped, anonymous ethical human tasks we ultimately have to face and explore from within and then call upon in the professional work of caring-healing. These are the deep tasks and human realities all health professionals face; this work ultimately involves human ontological caring competencies. Ultimately, this work requires turning toward what Stephen Mitchell noted as "the source and essence of all things, the luminous intelligence that shines from the depths of the human heart: the vital, immanent, subtle, radiant X . . . named by the ancients as 'unnamable reality'; 'that which causes everything to exist'" (1994:xiv). A turn toward "facing our humanity" and that of another, in the deep ethical sense meant by Levinas (1969), is the only way to sustain humanity across time; in this instance it is the source for sustaining Caring and Love and perhaps even the survival of the profession we know today as nursing.

By bringing attention to *Caritas Consciousness, Caritas Processes,* and refined Carative Factors, we are brought full circle—back to the deeply human and spirit-filled nature of professional nursing and an acknowledgment of the spiritual, mysterious, and sacred dimensions often silently residing in the margins of our work and our life. These dimensions cannot be ignored in a Philosophy and Science of Caring with an evolved *Caritas Consciousness* toward self and all of humanity. Continual spiritual growing and maturing are part of the journey of transpersonal awareness and *Caritas Consciousness Nursing.* It is a life-long journey.

> [W]e learn from one another how to be human by identifying our self with others, finding their dilemma in ourselves. What we all learn from this is self knowledge. The self we learn about . . . is every self. It is universal human self. We learn to recognize ourselves in others. [It] keeps alive our common humanity and avoids reducing self or other to the moral status of object. (Watson 1985:59–60)

ASSUMPTIONS OF A *CARITAS NURSE*: TRANSPERSONAL *CARITAS CONSCIOUSNESS* RELATIONSHIP

- The *Caritas Nurse* has a moral commitment to society and humanity. She or he is able to manifest an intentionality and *Caritas Consciousness* in relation with self and other to protect, enhance, promote, and preserve human dignity and wholeness.

- The *Caritas Nurse* affirms the subjective-spiritual significance of self and other while seeking to sustain caring in the midst of threat and despair, be it biological, institutional, or other.

- The *Caritas Nurse* honors an I-Thou relationship, not an I-It relationship.

- The *Caritas Nurse* seeks to recognize, honor, and accurately detect the spirit of the other through genuine presencing, being centered, available in the now-moment.

- Through actions, words, voice, nonverbal presence, thoughts, feelings, and full use of self, the *Caritas Nurse* connects with the other.

- The *Caritas* connection may occur through intentional yet authentic acts, movements, gestures, facial expressions, procedures, information giving, touch, voice, tone of voice, type of touch, soothing sounds, verbal expressions, and/or scientific-technical skills that communicate caring to the other. All these forms of professional and personal human communications and actions contribute to the transpersonal caring connection.

- The *Caritas Nurse* is not expected to have a transpersonal caring connection or caring moment with every patient. But *Caritas Consciousness* is held as a professional ideal to guide one's moral, ethical commitment and intentionality with each patient and sustain nursing's caring mission and covenant with society.

A CARING MOMENT

With every moment's light, may something beautiful be revealed to me, and become a part of who I am.

MARIANNE WILLIAMSON

A central component of the theory of transpersonal caring and *Caritas Consciousness,* already emphasized, is that it manifests in a given Now and becomes a part of both individuals who experience it. This is referred to in my work as a "Caring Moment."

The caring moment in-the-Now takes place when the nurse connects at a spirit-to-spirit level with another, beyond personality, physical appearance, disease, diagnosis, even presenting behavior; the nurse seeks to "see" who this spirit-filled person is as she or he "reads the field" in that instance. The *Caritas Nurse* in a caring moment is using all of his or her skill, knowledge, resources, and ways of knowing. In connecting this way, the moment becomes transcendent. This kind of moment is a focal experience in space and time, but a caring moment of connection in-the-Now transcends a sense of time and space; it has a field greater than the individuals who experience it. The connection goes beyond itself yet arises from itself in the moment, and it becomes part of the life history of each person and of the larger, complex pattern of life and the universe (Watson 1985).

HOLOGRAPHIC PREMISES OF
CARITAS CONSCIOUSNESS / RELATIONSHIP (WATSON 2005)

- The totality of *Caritas Consciousness* is contained and communicated in a single caring moment.

- The one-caring and the one-being-cared-for are connected with each other and the unified field of the universe to which we all belong.

- The *Caritas Consciousness* of the nurse is communicated to the other.

- *Caritas Consciousness* and the caring moment are transpersonal, in that they exist through time and space and are dominant over physical care alone.

- *Caritas Consciousness* transcends the moment; thus, it has possibilities that affect both people beyond the moment.

OTHER NURSING EXAMPLES CONSISTENT
WITH TRANSPERSONAL *CARITAS CONSCIOUSNESS*

Intentions remind us of what is important. . . . [I]ntention informs our choices and our actions. . . . [O]ur intentions serve as blueprints, allowing us to give shape and direction to our efforts . . . and our lives.

KABAT-ZINN AND KABAT-ZINN (1997:381)

[T]hinking related to intentionality connects with the concept of consciousness, energy. . . . [I]f our conscious intentionality is to hold [*Caritas*] thoughts that are caring, loving, open, kind, and receptive, in contrast to an intentionality to control, manipulate and have power over, the consequences will be significant . . . based on the different levels of consciousness . . . and the energy associated with the different thoughts.

WATSON (1999:121; [*CARITAS*] ADDED IN 2006)

Smith (1992) conducted an elaborate analysis of the extant caring literature using a Unitary Science lens. This perspective is consistent with the transpersonal dimensions discussed earlier, in that the unitary field of infinity is the context, transcending any given separate event and connecting all the parts to the whole. Her exploration of caring within this broader unitary field resulted in the identification and description of five constituents of caring:

1. Manifesting intention

2. Appreciating pattern

3. Attuning to dynamic flow

4. Experiencing the infinite

5. Inviting creative emergence.

Basically, Smith's analysis revealed shared themes across the different theoretical-philosophical writings on caring in nursing. When caring literature was explored within the unitary field of science, these were prominent features. They transcended the different authors and theories when lifted to a higher/deeper order of examination.

These dimensions and ways of seeing some of the universals of what manifests in a given caring moment can be considered transpersonal; that is, the concepts of manifesting intentions, appreciating pattern, attuning to dynamic flow (in the moment), inviting creative emergence, and experiencing the infinite are all operating as part of the holographic notions experienced in *Caritas Consciousness* and a Transpersonal Caring moment.

Notions of intentionality and its manifestation refer to a deep focus on a specific mental object of attention and awareness. Smith defined manifesting (caring) intentions as creating, holding, and expressing thoughts, images, feelings, beliefs, desires, will (purpose), and actions that affirm possibilities for human betterment or well-being (1992:14–28). Within the *Caritas* context, expressions of caring intentions could further include centering on the person in-the-now-moment; holding loving consciousness for preserving the person's wholeness, dignity, integrity; having reverence for what is emerging from the subjective inner processes; and approaching others with authentic presence, open to creative participation with infinity (Watson 2005).

While it is neither possible nor likely that these features will be present all the time, what happens in a caring moment does affect both parties, for better or for worse. The next section addresses the classic research of Halldorsdottir (1991), which helps us understand the for-better-or-for-worse outcomes of caring-noncaring for patients and nurses.

HALLDORSDOTTIR MODEL:
BIOCIDIC TO BIOGENIC (*CARITAS*) CARING

Halldorsdottir's (1991) clinical research led to a classification of nurse-patient relationships, based on the patients' experience, that allows us to grasp the continuum from uncaring to caring, which perhaps we can extend to *Caritas Consciousness* and add the continuum from non-healing to healing (Quinn et al. 2003).

- Type 1: Biocidic—life destroying (toxic, leading to anger, despair, and decreased well-being)

- Type 2: Biostatic—life restraining (cold, or patient treated as a nuisance)

- Type 3: Biopassive—life neutral (apathetic or detached)

- Type 4: Bioactive—life sustaining (classic nurse-patient relationship as kind, concerned, and benevolent)

- Type 5: Biogenic—life giving (life receiving).

The biogenic mode is closely aligned with notions of transpersonal and *Caritas Consciousness* in a caring-healing relationship. As Halldorsdottir put it:

> This [biogenic; transposed here as *Caritas* model] involves loving, benevolence, responsiveness, generosity, mercy and compassion. A truly life-giving presence offers the other interconnectedness and fosters spiritual freedom. It involves being open to persons and giving to the very heart of man [sic] as person, creating a relationship of openness and receptivity, yet always keeping a creative distance of respect and compassion. The truly life-giving or biogenic presence restores well-being and human dignity; it is a transforming, personal presence that deeply changes one. (Halldorsdottir 1991:44)

She continued, "For the recipient there is experienced an in-rush of compassion . . . like a river, and there is a transference of positive energy, strengthening, inspiring. . . . This life giving presence is greatly edifying for the soul of the other" (Halldorsdottir 1991:46).

This biogenic relationship parallels Watson's "transpersonal caring moment" (cited in Quinn et al. 2003) and its evolution here toward *Caritas Consciousness and Processes* as the basis for an authentic caring-healing relationship (Watson 2004a). For example, Halldorsdottir's research describes one patient as saying: "[T]he sense is somehow that your spirit and mine have met in the experience. And the whole idea [is] that there is somebody in the hospital who is *with* me, rather than working *on* me" (Halldorsdottir 1991:44).

FLORENCE NIGHTINGALE AS ORIGINAL THEORETICAL FOUNDATION FOR CARING/*CARITAS CONSCIOUSNESS* RELATIONSHIP

I would be remiss if I did not acknowledge the source and origin of caring-healing relationships in the ultimate sense that it is really nature that cures. Nightingale's well-known mandate is the common knowledge that the role of the nurse is to put the patient in the best condition for nature to act upon him or her (Nightingale 1969). It is assumed that we can now make new connections (from Nightingale forward to contemporary nursing literature to new science models): these caring, healing, loving relationships are natural; and, in Nightingale's model, such a relationship puts the person in the best condition for nature to act upon him or her. Indeed, in this *Caritas Nursing* model of Caring Science, it is the *Caritas Consciousness* within the relationship that guides professional actions, all of which contribute to healing and wholeness.

A recent research-guided document posited that "[t]he human to human relationship has the capacity to mediate a host of psychophysiological processes for better or for worse. . . . The biogenic or healing relationship assists in creating the conditions by which the innate tendency toward the emergence of healing is facilitated and enhanced in terms of renewal, order, increased coherence and transformation—the Haelan effect in Quinn's framework" (Quinn et al. 2003:A75). Likewise, one can posit the opposite; that is, patient-nurse relationships in which increased fear, anxiety, anger, despair, depression, and so on are present can be thought of as "unhealing" or, according to Halldorsdottir's research, biocidal or biocidic—the opposite of biogenic, life-giving, life-receiving relationships.

In addition to the nursing theoretical frameworks that support *Caritas Consciousness* in transpersonal caring-healing relationships, there is well-established "literature in psychoneuroimmunology, social support, love, and chaos and system theories which affirm[s] this perspective. Both social support and love have been shown to affect health status" (Quinn et al. 2003:A75). A theoretical statement that seems to connect all the notions put forth here about caring transpersonal relationships, *Caritas Consciousness*, evolving consciousness, healing, wholeness, natural process, love, and so on is summarized in a quote from Quinn and colleagues: "The healing relationship might be viewed as a type of critical social support, and as a particular kind of love, offered in moments of intense disequilibrium and vulnerability. It is, perhaps, the added energy in the system that allows the patient to emerge out of the chaos into a higher order—in other words, healing" (Quinn et al. 2003:A75).

REMINDERS

Concluding Summary Thoughts: *Caritas Consciousness* and the Transpersonal Caring Relationship

Carative Factor/*Caritas Process* 4: Developing and Sustaining an Authentic Caring Relationship (Watson 2005:185–186; reprinted with permission)

- Each thought and each choice we make carries spirit energy into our lives and those of others.

- Our [*Caritas*] consciousness, our intentionality, our presence, makes a difference for better or for worse.

- Calmness and mindfulness in a caring moment beget calmness and mindfulness.

- Caring and Love beget caring and love.

- Caring and compassionate acts of love beget healing for self and other.

- Transpersonal *Caritas Nursing* becomes transformative, liberating us to live and practice love and caring in our ordinary lives in non-ordinary ways.

Perennial Guidelines for Sustaining a *Caritas* Relationship

- Suspending role and status: honoring each person and her or his talents, gifts, and contributions as essential to the whole

- Speaking and listening without judgment, working from one's heart-centered space, working toward shared meaning and common values

- Listening with compassion and an open heart, without interrupting; listening to another's story as a healing gift of self

- Learning to be still, to center self, while welcoming and dwelling in silence for reflection, contemplation, and clarity

- Recognizing that transpersonal *Caritas* presence and practice transcend ego-self and connect us human-to-human, spirit-to-spirit to where our life and work are divided no more

- Honoring the reality that we are part of each other's journey; we are all on our own journey toward healing as part of the infinity of the human condition. When we work to heal ourselves, we contribute to healing the whole.

RELATIONSHIP-CENTERED CARING MODEL

An educational template for Teaching Relationship-Centered Caring to all health professions was developed by the Pew Fetzer Task Group on Relationship-Centered Caring (1994). The Pew Fetzer Report (PFR) on Relationship-Centered Care (1994), a national project in which I participated, identified a set of knowledge, skills, and values associated with the health practitioner–caring relationship at several levels:

- Practitioner's relationship with self
- Practitioner-to-patient relationship
- Practitioner-to-community relationship
- Practitioner-to-practitioner relationship.

This information can be incorporated into educational curricula and clinical learning experiences for all health care practitioners.

Table 8.1 Practitioner Relationship with Self (modified from PFR 1994:30)

Area: Self-Relationship	Knowledge	Skills	Values
Self-awareness, self-knowledge, self-growth; developing a helping-trusting-caring relationship with self	Knowledge of self; understanding self as resource/healing agent for self/other Knowledge of selected "Carative Factors" Knowledge of *Caring moment and Transpersonal Caring-Healing* processes	Reflect on self/work; ability to *be authentically present*; cultivation of sensitivity to self and other; enabling hope and faith "Ontological competencies"	Importance of self-awareness/self-caring/self-growth Honoring spiritual dimensions in caring process Honoring unity of Being; Honoring mind-body-spirit as One
Patient experiences with and meaning of health-illness, healing, caring needs	Role of family, culture, community Multiple components of health Multiple threats and contributors to health as dimensions of one's reality	Recognize patient's life story and its inner and outer meanings for person View health and illness as part of self-growth and human development, a potential existential turning point	Appreciation of patient as whole person Appreciation of patient's story and beliefs and practices
Developing and maintaining caring relationship with self and other	Understanding threats to the integrity of relationship (e.g., power, control inequalities) Understanding destructive non-caring; potential for abuse, conflict	Attend fully to patient, with active listening, full presence Accept and respond to distress in patient and self Respond to moral and ethical challenges	Respect for patient's dignity, uniqueness, and integrity (mind-body-spirit unity) Respect for self-control, self-knowledge, self-healing potential, self-determination

continued on next page

Table 8.1—continued

Area: Self-Relationship	Knowledge	Skills	Values
		Facilitate trust, faith, and hope	Respect for person's own inner power and spiritual-mental-physical processes for accessing healer within
		Cultivate personal/professional practices for self-growth, insight, reflection	
Effective and constructive caring communication	Elements of effective communication and being present and in relation	Listen, *Hear*	Valuing one's intuition, inner knowing; open, nonjudgmental, compassionate
		Teaching-Learning	
		Accept patient's emotions and knowledge	

Tables 8.1–8.4 can serve as an educational-practice guide for developing knowledge, skills, and values for Relationship-Centered Caring. Table 8.2 outlines a framework for Relationship-Centered Caring. It encompasses the Practitioner Relationship with Self as a foundational starting point and extends to the Practitioner-Patient Relationship.

The next sections incorporate Practitioner-to-Community Relationships and Practitioner-to Practitioner Relationships. The goal is to outline a foundational model for education and practice that will prepare and generate future individual and communities of caring-healing practitioners—practitioners working together to serve the complex matrix of individuals' needs in health, illness, and caring-healing processes and outcomes while also continually cultivating and deepening biogenic relationships with self and other.

Practitioner-to-Community Relationship

The practitioner-to-community relationship acknowledges that caring and relationship cannot be based solely on an individualistic model of caring but makes explicit that caring begins with self and radiates out from self to other, to family, community, planet Earth, even to the cosmos, affecting the entire infinity field of humanity (Levinas 1969; Watson 2005). This notion of caring that extends beyond the individual is grounded in the Latin word *Caritas*, conveying caring at a deeper level than conventional thinking. *Caritas* conveys connections between caring and love, allowing for a new form of deep transpersonal caring for self and other. This relationship between caring and love connotes inner processes and extends to nature and the larger universe (Watson 2004a:13).

Caritas-to-Communitas. In extending caring to a model of *Caritas,* or *"clinical Caritas"* (Watson 2004a), the underlying values are made explicit. This notion of *Caritas*/deep caring is consistent with Nightingale's sense of "calling" into nursing as a commitment with a professional and personal covenantal ethic of compassionate human service guided by an "altruistic-humanistic value system" (Watson 1985). It is acknowledged in this extended framework that caring is a phenomenon that is to be cherished; it is very fragile, delicate, and

Table 8.2 Practitioner-to-Patient Relationship (modified from PFR 1994:30)

Area	Knowledge	Skills	Values
Self-awareness	Knowledge of self: understand self as source for others	Reflect on self and work	Importance of self-awareness, self-care, self-growth
Patient experience of health and illness	Role of family, culture, community development; multiple components of health; multiple threats and contributors	Recognize patient's life story and its meaning View health and illness as part of human development	Appreciation of patient as a whole person Appreciation of patient's life story and the meaning of the health-illness condition
Developing and maintaining caring relationship	Understand threats to the integrity of the relationship; e.g., power inequalities, potential for conflict and abuse	Attend fully to patient Accept and respond to distress in patient and self Respond to moral and ethical challenges Facilitate hope, trust, and faith	Respect patient's dignity, uniqueness, and integrity (mind-body-spirit unity) Respect self-determination Respect person's own power and self-healing processes
Effective communication	Elements of effective communication	Listen, impart information, Learn Facilitate learning of others Promote and accept patient's emotions	Importance of being open and non-judgmental

precious, requiring attention and cultivation to sustain. "When caring and love come together to serve humankind, we discover and affirm that nursing and caring-healing work is more than just a job, but a life-giving and life-receiving [biogenic] career for a lifetime of growth and learning" (Watson 2004a:13).

As this model becomes more explicit, we are increasingly able to integrate the past with the present and the future. Such maturity and evolution require (consistent with the PFR) "transforming self and those we serve, including our institutions and the profession itself" (Watson 2004a:13). As we more publicly and professionally assert a model of caring relationship, grounded in notions of *Caritas* and biogenic/transpersonal dimensions of caring for self and other, we locate our self and our profession within a new emerging cosmology of caring and loving as part of healing relationships. Through this shift, we call forth a sense of reverence and sacredness with respect to self, other, and all living things, thus invoking and transposing *Caritas* to extend to *Communitas* in thinking and actions as a new and deep form of Practitioner-to-Community Relationships and an evolving relational, eco-caring worldview.

Communitas. This interconnection between *Caritas and Communitas* makes explicit that we belong to a shared humanity and are connected with each other. In this way, we share our collective humanity across time and space and are bound together in the infinite universal field that holds the totality of life itself.

The Pew Fetzer Report (PFR 1994:27) reminded us more concretely that individuals belong simultaneously to multiple communities formed by neighborhoods, cultures, work groups, and circumstances. Moreover, a person hospitalized for an extended period becomes part of the hospital community:

> Through their relationships with—and memberships in—various
> communities, practitioners have a voice and substantial responsi-
> bilities in the work that focuses on the cultural and environmen-
> tal determinants of health. They need to understand the broad
> social, political and cultural, economic, and policy determinants
> of health; recognize and act in accordance with the values, norms,

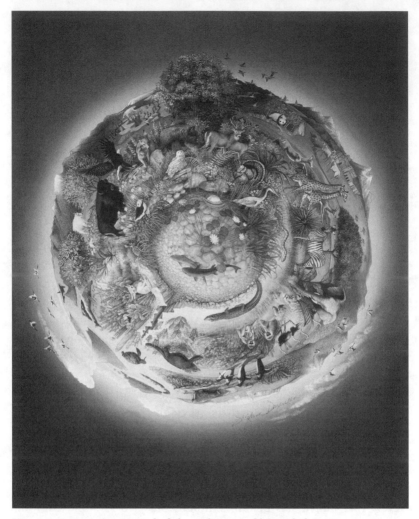

Figure 9. An artist's portrayal of the evolving worldview shift to an eco-caring cosmology, an inner and outer vision of wholeness, and the connectedness of all life on Earth. © Suzanne Duranceau 1990. Reprinted with permission.

social and health concerns of the community; develop a sense of community responsibility; be able to recognize harmful elements within the community; and work to change harmful aspects of the community to improve its health. (PFR 1994:27)

The attention to cultivating practitioner-to-community relationships is based further on an ethic and ethos of shared humanity, which reminds us that we learn to be more human by seeing our self in the other and vice versa, realizing that one level of humanity reflects back on the other. This ethic and ethos is located within an emerging cosmology referred to as Unitary Consciousness (Watson 1999), noting that everything in the universe is connected, not separate and disconnected. Thus, we learn to be more open, more available, more present to the wonders of life itself, bonding us through the very breath of life, honoring the fact that we share the air we breathe. *Caritas* and *Communitas* define an emerging global ethic of caring-healing through relationships, belonging, and connectedness, which helps us restore the sacred in the midst of everyday existence and our relationship to all living things.

The knowledge, skills, and values in which practitioners need to effectively participate as part of their work with communities fall into four areas in the Pew Fetzer framework (PFR 1994:31):

1. The meaning of community (extended here to include the concept of *Caritas-Communitas*)

2. The multiple contributors to health and illness within the community

3. Developing and maintaining relationships with the community (at multiple levels of awareness of community)

4. Effective community-based care.

These categories can serve as a curricular framework and guide for comprehending community in a broad sense. However, the nature, definitions, and meaning of community are constantly changing in society and the world. Indeed, even our worldview is shifting when considering community in its broadest, universal sense.

Table 8.3 summarizes the categories of practitioner-to-community relationships identified/modified from the Pew Fetzer Report.

Developing and sustaining a deeper understanding of community—within both a concrete, local, and immediate sense and a universal *Communitas* sense—form the foundation for effective caring. It

Table 8.3 Practitioner-to-Community Relationships (modified from PFR 1994:34)

Area	Knowledge	Skills	Values
Meaning of community (extending notion of *Caritas-Communitas*)	Various models of community Myths and perceptions about community Perspectives from diverse disciplines Dynamic change, demographic, political, and so on	Learn continually Participate actively in community development Engage in dialogue with others	Respect integrity Communitarian ethic Honor belongingness with other; unitary awareness Respect for human-cultural diversity/dignity of shared humanity
Multiple contributors to health within the community	History of community, land use, migration, occupations; their effect on health Physical, social, occupational environments; their effect on health; influencing external-internal forces	Critically assess relationship of health care providers to community health Assess community environmental health Policy/worldview implications	Affirm relevance of universality of a communitarian view of determinants of health Affirm value of health policy
Develop and maintain community relationships	History of practitioner-community relationships Isolation of health care team from community at large	Communicate ideas Listen openly Empower self and others; learn Facilitate learning of others Participate in community development Engage in caring and social action	Be open-minded Be honest regarding limits of health/medical science Responsibility to contribute health-caring relational expertise
Effective community-based care	Various types of care, formal and informal Effects of institution on care Positive effects of continuity of care/caring/relationship/connectedness	Collaborate in caring relationship with other individuals and organizations Work as member of team, healing community Instrument of change	Respect for community leadership Commit to work for change Help create communities of caring-healing, compassionate human service

is in recognizing, honoring, and explicating incorporation of a caring-communitarian ethic and ethos into our practice models that we help sustain individual and community. Further, it is by giving expanded attention to community relations that we bring forth our belongingness, our connectedness, and our shared human conditions. It is through this awareness and awakening that we cultivate more compassion, wisdom, and skills for caring and for relationships, individually and collectively. It is through this awakening that we become agents and instruments for a moral community of caring. Thus, in this model we are ever more leaning and learning to evolve toward a global ethic of *Caritas-Communitas* as a worldview as well as a professional relationship-centered, caring practice model—a model that invites, inspires, and helps sustain our humanity and our world.

Practitioner-to-Practitioner Relationships

As relationship-centered caring becomes more central to health care, and as practitioners awaken to the shift in health care from curing to healing, it becomes evident that caring-healing relationships between and among practitioners themselves are critical. Without a caring team that works together to promote harmony and healing among themselves and those they serve, the entire system is affected. Thus, the quality of relationships among all members of a health community affects the capacity of everyone within it. The ability to create and sustain practitioner-to-practitioner relationships affects each practitioner's ability and conditions to care for self, patient, systems, communities, and, ultimately, society. Forming caring-healing practitioner communities allows for incorporating and honoring the diverse yet shared knowledge, skills, and values each profession and practitioner brings to the community. The practitioner-to-practitioner emphasis values the individual and collective talents and gifts.

Practitioner-to-practitioner relationship building begins by affirming the shared values, missions, tasks, goals, and talents of the team (PFR 1994:35). The same caring relationship skill set and consciousness are required among team members as the one needed between patient and practitioner; that is, being present, honoring the unique subjective world of the other, openly listening with intent to hear the other's point of view, and communicating congruence and differences effectively. The need exists to confront disagreements and misunderstandings directly in such a way that conflict is resolved in a constructive manner rather than ignored and allowed to grow.

It is a given that different professions and backgrounds among practitioners will manifest different traditions of knowledge and practices. Each will also bring different skills and talents that can be encompassed and embraced to round out the entire team, recognizing that everyone has something unique to offer and making the effect more wholesome, complete, and whole. Affirming and valuing diversity among the team are necessary. Practitioners can learn from each other about the healing approaches of other professions and cultures. Together, they can learn to honor and respect and appreciate the mix of talents, to know the value of others' work and continually learn from others, including professional, lay, and indigenous healing traditions and practices. Awakening to the importance of creating and sustaining a community of caring-healing practitioners can be the foundation for transforming sick care into health and healing for all. Once awakened to this new reality that cooperation and community/*Communitas* are the basis of true health care, it becomes the ethical-moral responsibility of professionals at all levels to work from this caring center. Then we all learn true humility, to let go of ego, to grow beyond personal/professional, limited—and sometimes arrogant—agendas. We learn how to value, give, and receive mutual trust, support, kindness, patience, and emotional regard for self and other. In addition, we learn to "exhibit a capacity for grace, which represents an attitude of decency, thoughtfulness, and generosity of spirit toward [self] and others" (PFR 1994:36).

In addition, we each learn humility by acknowledging that no one discipline, person, or professional works alone or has all the knowledge, skills, values, and experience necessary for deeply human caring and healing work. Thus, this work takes on human dimensions that can be celebrated, cultivated, and embraced instead of controlled by attempts to fix and blame others and by perceiving each individual practitioner as essentially alone, performing isolated events. Nothing is isolated in this model; rather, we are all connected and interdependent.

Caritas-Communitas-Love and Caring Human-to-Human Connections become paramount.

Table 8.4 includes the areas of knowledge, skills, and values associated with practitioner-to-practitioner caring-healing relationships, identified by the Pew Fetzer Report (PFR 1994:36).

An understanding of all these dimensions and vicissitudes of relationship and caring is the basis for creating a more integrated model of caring-healing, of *Caritas* to *Communitas*. The relationship practitioners form with self, patient, community, and other practitioners is critical and requires balanced attention to transform education and practice as well as the practitioners themselves, whether students or skilled clinicians (PFR 1994:37). Subsequent chapters will continue to unfold knowledge, skills, and values that will deepen and strengthen relationship-centered caring as a moral, philosophical, and practical foundation for nursing and health care practices.

Table 8.4 Areas of Knowledge, Skills, and Values for Practitioner-to-Practitioner Relationships (modified from PFR 1994:36)

Area	Knowledge	Skills	Values
Self-awareness	Knowledge of self in relation to other; connectedness and unity worldview	Reflect on self-in-relation Learn continually See other in self and vice versa; shared humanity	Self-awareness Caritas/Communitas as moral model for caring-healing relationships
Traditions of knowledge, diverse professions	Healing approaches of various professions, lay and indigenous Healing approaches across cultures Historical inequities/power	Derive meaning from others' work Learn from experience within healing community	Affirm and value diversity and share human connections beyond role, professional background
Build teams and moral communities of caring	Different perspectives on teams, conflict resolution, communication Listen openly Learn cooperatively See self in other	Communicate effectively	Affirm and honor mission, diversity, shared connections, caring community as ethic
Working dynamics of teams, groups, organizations	Perspectives on team dynamics from various sciences, including caring sciences/social science	Share responsibility Collaborate with others Work cooperatively Resolve conflict	Openness to others' ideas Humility Mutual trust, empathy, support Capacity for grace

From **CARATIVE FACTOR 5:** *Promotion and Acceptance of the Expression of Positive and Negative Feelings* to **CARITAS PROCESS 5:** *Being Present to, and Supportive of, the Expression of Positive and Negative Feelings** *

This Carative Factor / *Caritas Process* extension is embedded in discussions in previous chapters of the transpersonal and the nature and differences between, for example, a noncaring relationship (biocidic) and a healing relationship (biogenic-transpersonal) (Halldorsdottir 1991). This factor may not need to be discussed separately, since it is inherent and intrinsically related to the development of an authentic trusting, caring relationship.

However, because this dimension and dynamic of relationship building is so basic, it can be, and often is, taken for granted, not even recognized or attended to in professional practice. Thus, I continue to explore it here.

---

* As a connection with deeper spirit of self and the one-being-cared-for: listening to, holding another person's story.

It is through being present to and allowing constructive expression of all feelings that we create a foundation for trust and caring. When one is able to hold the tears or fears of another without being threatened or turning away, that is an act of healing and caring.

When one is able, through his or her *Caritas Consciousness*, to enter into the life space of another, connecting with the inner subjective life world of emotions and thoughts, one is connecting with the deeper spirit of self and other. This is the foundation for a transpersonal caring moment and a healing relationship.

It is an established fact that thoughts and emotions play a central role in people's experiences and behavior. Knowledge of psychology, psychodynamics, and psychiatry, as well as common life experiences, helps us understand and comprehend the power and importance of emotions.

Early research in social psychology has shown that behavior and decision making, especially in conflict-laden situations, are both rational and quasi-rational (emotional-affective). This connection of emotional components has been theoretically and empirically validated in social science and behavioral science literature. It has long been acknowledged that emotions constitute one of the primary motivations for humans. Thus, it can be understood that intellectual understanding of information and the emotional understanding of that same information can be and usually are quite different. This disjunction has commonly been referred to in the social psychology literature as affective-cognitive dissonance. An individual usually seeks consistency between disparate thoughts and emotions when such dissonance occurs; consistency is sought with the intent to find meaning, harmony, and balance in one's life and world.

When inconsistency or dissonance continues or escalates, one becomes more anxious, fearful, confused, stressed. Inconsistency and emotional-cognitive dissonance can affect attitudes, understandings, and behavior. In an interpersonal relationship, and in situations related to health and illness, it is often the emotional aspect at the feeling level that explains whether people are able to communicate smoothly, hear each other, listen, establish rapport, and so on. This dynamic of understanding human behavior is foundational to building and sustaining a helping-trusting-caring relationship.

Professionals in all fields have to grasp and appreciate this basic fact of our shared humanity if we are to effectively relate and communicate, one to another, in ways that are "healthogenic" or "biogenic." What is often the most troubling in relationship building is someone reacting negatively, when the other person's feelings seem "nonrational," disruptive, threatening, angry, or inappropriate for the situation. These instances are precisely when presence and openness and acceptance come into play in a most essential, sensitive way.

The first *Caritas Process*: Loving-Kindness and Equanimity, allows the person to have his or her feelings, both positive and negative. In allowing and facilitating their expression, the nurse is contributing to the process of both honoring and accepting one's feelings while also creating an awareness whereby the feelings are able to move through the individual for release in a constructive way. The person is thus helped to empty out, releasing passing feelings that were contributing to confusion, fear, anger, and so on. It is known in psychoanalytical and everyday experiences that an awareness of one's feelings may eliminate some of the irrationality of emotional outbursts and give one more self-control over thoughts and behavior. For example, if someone is made aware of his or her feelings, it is easier to accept them, understand them, and see how they are influencing behavior. There is no right or wrong to feelings; they just are.

It is how we accept, honor, and respond to our feelings that makes the difference in our emotional and cognitive life world. Once we are able to honor our feelings, to give ourselves permission to feel, we are made more aware of the feelings. Then we can better understand the deeper emotions and situation that may have triggered the specific feelings.

Eventually, we understand that feelings are universal, that there is no such thing as a good or bad feeling. Everyone has feelings. That realization alone may free the person, allowing for equanimity, forgiveness, and gentleness toward self. Feelings come and go, but we realize that we are not our feelings. Then one is free to respond to the situation more clearly, more appropriately, even with a sense of loving-kindness and compassion. Thus, the expression of feelings is a healing act in itself.

The process of being with another in a nonjudgmental way as that individual expresses his or her feelings generates a mutual trust and understanding. This process serves as a core foundation that sustains the authenticity of a caring relationship and affirms the shared humanity of both individuals in that moment.

The literature has established that a change in any emotion, behavior, or cognition may cause a change in the other two. The affective component of an attitude is said to be that aspect that is emotionally satisfying; this view suggests that a person seeks consistency between emotions and thoughts, that emotions serve a need as humans seek to maintain a balance between and among thoughts, feelings, and behavior.

The earlier work of Yalom (1975) supports the importance of this factor/process. In his classic clinical studies with patients in group therapy, he found that when asked to recall a single critical incident that served as a turning point for them, the incident most often reported was a sudden expression of strong negative feelings (e.g., hatred or anger). The common characteristics of the critical incident were:

- The person expressed a strong negative emotion, which was new for him or her.
- The feared or fantasized catastrophe associated with the expression of the negative feelings did not occur.
- Reality testing ensued in which the person realized that the feeling expressed was inappropriate in intensity or direction or that the avoidance of the expression of the feeling was irrational (the person may or may not have gained insight into or psychodynamic knowledge of the source of the feelings).
- The person was enabled to interact and to explore more deeply.

In this same work, the expression of strong positive feelings had almost the same therapeutic outcome as the expression of negative feelings. For example, the common critical incidents related to the expression of positive emotion were:

- The person was able to express a strong positive emotion, which was unusual for him or her.

- The feared rejection or fantasized catastrophe did not occur; there was no rejection, deriding, or damage to others by the person displaying the positive feelings.

- The person discovered a previously unknown part of self, which resulted in a new dimension in relationships with self and others.

These findings help validate what is already common knowledge: that helping another to nonjudgmentally express positive and negative feelings without feeling defensive or threatened by rejection and criticism is therapeutic. The *Caritas Consciousness Nurse* is aware and confident enough to permit another to risk expressing feelings that otherwise would be threatening. In turn, the caring relationship moves to a deeper, more honest, authentic level that is necessary for the practice of the philosophy and science of caring.

Authentically hearing and accepting another person's story not only helps that person express his or her feelings, it becomes a healing act in itself, a healing gift to others. The nurse in a given moment may be the only person who is able to hear and receive another person's story and emotions, thus helping that person find deeper meaning in his or her situation. The *Caritas Consciousness Nurse* may be the only person who seeks to "see" and "hear" the spirit-filled person behind the emotions. This process can lead to more self-knowledge, self-control, self-love, and self-caring possibilities.

Finally, if feelings, both positive and negative, can and do change thoughts and influence one's relationship with self and other, the practice of caring must be systematically attentive to people's feelings. *Caritas*

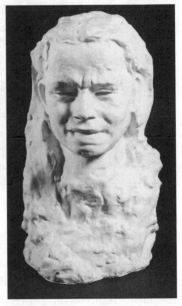

Figure 10. La Pleureuse, *by Auguste Rodin. Collection, The Denver Art Museum.*

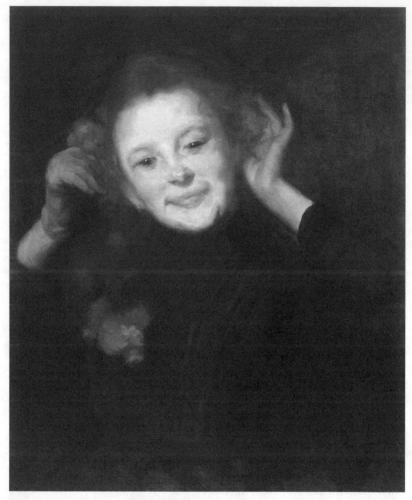

Figure 11. Young Girl with Flowers, *by Eugène Carrière. Collection, The Denver Art Museum.*

Consciousness, with its intellectual, philosophical, and experiential knowing of this common human dynamic and how it affects all aspects of caring relationships, brings this Carative Factor / *Caritas Process* from the background of our professional practices to the foreground.

CHAPTER TEN

From **CARATIVE FACTOR 6:** *Systematic Use of the Scientific Problem-Solving Method for Decision Making* *to* **CARITAS PROCESS 6:** *Creative Use of Self and All Ways of Knowing as Part of the Caring Process; Engage in the Artistry of* Caritas Nursing

Professional nursing involves systematic logic, along with imagination and creativity. The nursing process is acknowledged as a systematic process that guides nurses' decision making. However, it is important to acknowledge that a more expanded Caring/*Caritas Process* is not a systematic, linear process as it is often made out to be and as originally presented in my 1979 book. Indeed, of all the Carative Factors in the original book, this one has changed the most during my growth, maturity, and evolution over the years. In 1979 I had just completed my PhD—I was idealistic, naive, and enamored with research and scientific methods as the basis for advancing nursing science and practice. The evolved *Caritas Nurse* celebrates the caring process as a creative, intuitive, aesthetic, ethical, personal, even spiritual process, as well as a professional empirical-technical process.

However, while nursing scholarship within a *Caritas Model* has matured, Janice Muff's earlier (1988) critique of nursing from an outside lens unfortunately still lingers in educational and practice mindsets; that is, authoritarianism has a strong tradition throughout nursing education and practice cultures. Her research found that nursing instructors often believe and teach "that there is only one right way to do things—their way." As she viewed it, nursing creates self-imposed restrictions on itself. For example, despite nursing faculty's rhetoric of developing autonomous professionals, agents of change, leaders, and so on, nursing students are often rewarded more for obedience and conformity than for assertiveness, questioning, and differences of opinion (Watson 1999).

The often arbitrary, linear "nursing process" to which nurses have historically subscribed as a formal procedure is too often presented as a truism and the only way to problem solve, when in reality it does not work that way. In fact, the nursing process is merely a common problem-solving process that has been renamed and relabeled "nursing process." These identity and boundary structures create false boundaries and a false impression that nursing has some special approach to problem solving (Muff 1988).

Nurses have a history of working from set roles and functions, of fixed ways of being and doing, without those methods necessarily being scientific or scholarly. In spite of advanced education, scholarly practices, and role changes, today, in its own way, a robotic tendency has emerged in the fast-paced institutional system, reinforcing the old tendency to adhere to rigid technical mind-sets and medical-techno-cure institutional demands. This habitual institutional mind-set happens without awareness, without pausing to critique, without bringing one's full consciousness and intentionality to bear on the use of the available expanded knowledge, values, and human dynamics necessary for a reflective practice model that embraces the best of both science and art.

A glimpse into conventional nursing and nurse detachment in an effort to be "professional" and in some instances "scientific," which is separate from a caring-healing relationship, is captured in Sylvia Plath's classic poem "Tulips," which was written after she was hospitalized.

"Tulips" I, from *Ariel* by Sylvia Plath*

The tulips are too excitable, it is winter here.
Look how white everything is, how quiet, how snowed in.
I am learning peacefulness, lying by myself quietly
As the light lies on these white walls, this bed, these hands.
I am nobody; I have nothing to do with explosions.
I have given my name and my day-clothes up to the nurses
And my history to the anaesthetist and my body to surgeons.
They have propped my head between the pillow and the sheet-cuff.
Like an eye between two white lids that will not shut.
Stupid pupil, it has to take everything in.
The nurses pass and pass, they are no trouble,
They pass the way gulls pass inland in their white caps.
Doing things with their hands, one just the same as another,
So it is impossible to tell how many there are.

My body is a pebble to them, they tend it as water
Tends to the pebbles it must run over, smoothing them gently.
They bring me numbness in their bright needles, they bring me sleep.
Now I have lost myself I am sick of baggage—
My patent leather overnight case like a black pillbox,
My husband and child smiling out of the family photo,
Their smiles catch onto my skin, little smiling hooks.
I have let things slip, a thirty-year-old cargo boat
Stubbornly hanging on to my name and address.
They have swabbed me clear of my loving associations.
Scared and bare on the green plastic-pillowed trolley
I watched my tea-set, my bureaus of linen, my books
Sink out of sight, and the water went over my head.
I am a nun now; I have never been so pure.

I emphasize that science and human values go together. A Caring Science makes explicit that a difference exists among data, information, and knowledge. Information is not knowledge; knowledge alone does not mean understanding; even understanding, in isolation, does not necessarily include insight, reflection, and wisdom. *Caritas*

* © 1962 by Ted Hughes, by permission of Harper & Row Publishers, Inc.

Processes seek information, knowledge, understanding, and wisdom (Watson 2005).

The ultimate goals of nursing care, Caring Science, and research are to deliver quality, humane care. The method for delivering quality, humane scientific and artistic caring-healing requires the formal use of a creative problem-solving process and the systematic use of cognitive, rational logic, along with all ways of knowing. Caring Science honors diverse sources of knowledge, multiple methodologies, and expanded views of a relational ontology. It includes caring ethics as well as empirical evidence: the art and science of caring, healing, and health. The development and practices of nursing and Caring Science are sophisticated and complex. Nursing is constantly maturing, advancing, and developing in its scholarly orientation toward caring practices and research.

RECONSIDERING EVIDENCE-BASED PRACTICE

Earlier in nursing's history, there was strict adherence to a linear view of the nursing process; today, there is a great focus on "evidence-based practice." Evidence remains an ambiguous term and phenomenon, in that "medical evidence differs from reflection from a phenomenological concept of evidence gleaned from personal story" (Martinsen 2006:11). Kari Martinsen (2006), in her latest theoretical work from Norway, draws on Logstrup's view of evidence as "the evident": the insights and existential questions emerging from within the narrative expression of one's life philosophy, that which can be trusted.

Evidence-based medicine (EBM), which has influenced evidence-based nursing (EBN), is derived from clinically controlled studies and statistical concepts as the empirical-technical basis for a system of knowledge. The origin is in epidemiological and general statistical population-based research. As Martinsen (2006:123) put it: "How does this kind of evidence relate to judgment [wisdom], which is so important in all research and practical work?"

In other words, we are invited to reflect upon and analyze, as well as critique, issues. It is important to ask questions, such as how and where do a philosophy of caring and healing and a philosophical orientation toward what Martinsen (2006:123) calls "life possibilities in a health profession" fit in a culture currently dominated by evidence-based medical thinking?

Reminding us of different forms of evidence, Martinsen references Finnish nursing scholar Katie Eriksson (1999). Together, they point out that "linguistically, the meaning of evidence is to see and to gain insight into; the word 'evidence' is related to 'knowing,' which again may mean to attend to, to become familiar with, to experience, and based on this, [to] reach an indisputable certainty regarding some issue" (Martinsen 2006:123). Thus, evidence has strong ties to the obvious, the palpable, the incontestable, the distinct and clear, as well as to the proof of natural events.

Therefore, such expanded and deepened notions of evidence and seeing relate to theory in the Latin/Greek word sense, in that the word *theoria* can be translated as "to see." When these notions are linked, we focus on gaining insight into, attending to, knowing, experiencing, judging: using all ways of knowing. Thus, these notions give a much wider and deeper meaning to "adequacy of evidence," beyond simply proving or measuring or validating an empirical fact.

In this more expanded and broader view of evidence, we can seek to distinguish between complete (adequate) evidence and incomplete (inadequate) evidence (Martinsen 2006:124). Further, in clarifying this line of thinking, we can begin to unravel certain forms of evidence, such as subject matter, some experiences, situations, phenomena, and even pre-scientific, pre-conscious notions, as well as objective external givens, facts, and so forth. Each form of evidence may yield different forms of knowledge pertaining to certain situations and objects of analysis: inner or outer phenomena. One form of evidence may not conform to another form of evidence needed for adequate decision making; congruence between different forms of evidence is necessary to understand human experiences in this living human-environmental field of complexities, ambiguities, and unknowns.

While it is critical to have evidence and scientific-technical, empirical knowledge for professional practice, the phenomenon of nursing evidence has to be expanded and deepened in the fullest sense of the word for professional care to occur; thus, the notion and process of evidence need to be critiqued, discussed, and unraveled for the best practice.

In reality, neither the nurse nor the physician can take a single piece of "evidence," a single research finding, a single theoretical or empirical fact, and translate any or all of it into a single, simplistic, systematic, scientific, evidentiary, linear problem-solving process in a given patient care situation. It is not possible to do so. Human beings are too complex for such a linear response to evidence to be effective.

In addition, it is important to remind ourselves once again that "evidence" takes many forms and that there is a difference between data and information, knowledge, understanding, and wisdom. That is, a loose datum is not coherent information; information is not the same as knowledge; and knowledge alone without reflection, processing, and integration into specific and complex situations is not wisdom. So, having information related to evidence per se, without translating that information into knowledge associated with the complexity of human life and the current world situation, is not necessarily useful. A wise *Caritas* practitioner seeks to integrate necessary "evidence" at multiple levels with the wise clinical judgment necessary for addressing individual people with individual life stories and circumstances: integrating practitioner and person-patient-family.

ASKING NEW QUESTIONS ABOUT "EVIDENCE"

Nursing is at a dramatic turning point at this point in the twenty-first century. If nursing is to evolve and mature as a discipline and a distinct caring profession, it is appropriate to critique and raise new questions and to explore a variety of discourses about what counts as evidence. Thus, there are different ways of validating or testing situations with regard to what counts as evidence.

Does one's clinical judgment count as evidence? Does the nurse's dissonance between affective and cognitive impressions and among rational, quasi-rational, affective impressions count as evidence? (See Chapter 9.)

Does Nursing Theory count as evidence? Do personal perceptions, knowledge, values, ethics, intuition, and perceptions count? These questions need to be raised in the field of Caring Science if nursing is to avoid jumping on a restrictive linear process in considering a knee-jerk approach to evidence—an approach that is linear, limiting, technical, and empirical. Such data-related evidence can be fed into a computer, but that can result in eliminating the human factor, the ethical-value factor, and the complex, professional caring process as parts of a complete, wise clinical experience.

As Martinsen put it (2006:125): "To examine the experience of the world with which I indubitably communicate is different from accounting for a statistical relation or presenting a proof. Different demands . . . must be made to that which is understood as evident, depending on what one wants to know about or make apparent."

In a mature model for incorporating evidence, empirical-technical-scientific knowledge and informed moral practice come together in a given moment, drawing upon all of one's knowledge, experiences, judgment, wisdom, and skills in that moment. The complexity of the whole becomes foreground; the evidence and the problem-solving/nursing process are the background that informs the foreground of *Caritas Nursing*.

Martinsen (2006:126) warns us against making an "instrumentalistic mistake"; that is, giving an instrumental, rational reason a privileged position as normative for human communication or making "scientific-technical knowledge into a model for human actions of an . . . ethical character." A strictly utilitarian reason cannot be the sole basis of decision making and use of evidence. She considers doing so a transgression of the caring ethic and professional responsibility.

Thus, all forms of evidence need to have a voice so no single form of evidence is excluded at the expense of another. Martinsen (2006) makes a case for the use of what I think of as authentic dialogue, or what she notes as equal footing, equal voice, in which all parties have a conversation to attain evident insights. Such a situation entails facing an issue or a problem in the highest light, creating freedom between and among all the parties, all the voices of evidence, even though the focus and tasks may differ.

CARITAS PROCESS

A *Caritas Process* critiques a superficial interpretation of both Nursing Process and Evidence-Based Practice. A *Caritas Process* honors the creative, individualized, caring process that draws upon all ways of knowing/being/doing. The *Caritas Process* integrates and is informed by the best sources of evidence, within a horizon of knowledge that embraces theory, ethics, values, and the best personal-professional, empirical-technical clinical judgment and decision making available at the moment.

The complexity of decision making and acting within *Caritas Processes* requires critical thinking, clarity of rationale, and use of scientific evidence; but it also demands a focus and an orientation that make explicit the multifaceted creative, integrative, critical thinking necessary for engaging in a systematic, synthesized problem-solving focus for an individualized, living-breathing patient care situation. Such a *Caritas Process* calls upon full use of self. All knowledge is honored as valuable; it is accessed and processed in making the best caring decision in the given situation. This process thus cannot be framed as an absolutist framework—it is relative to the individual nurse, patient, family, team, and creative processing, integrating, and reflecting; to the dialogues and conversation required in this specific situation.

Within the *Caritas* model, all knowledge counts as evidence; all knowledge and perceptions are processed, reflected upon as valuable. This complex process is not strictly scientific or fully empirically based but calls upon creative moral imagination as well as a systematic problem-solving approach. The *Caritas Nurse* honors the best sources of all known evidence, inviting inquisitive risk taking, critiquing, and exploratory approaches not stifled by a limited, one-way approach.

The *Caritas Nurse* aspires to be present in-the-Now-moments, to read the gestalt of the emerging field, and to respond by drawing upon all ways of knowing/being/doing. The hoped-for direction is toward moral wisdom and what Martinsen (2006:132) refers to as "seeing with the heart's eye," inviting us into a new, expansive space as to what kind of self one should realize and "how should I live my life" as a *Caritas Nurse* and person.

PHILOSOPHICAL PERSPECTIVE
FOR CARING SCIENCE: *CARITAS PROCESSES*

A strict absolutist mind-set toward science, knowledge, evidence, and nursing processes often conflicts with other ways of knowing, expanded views of science, and the dissonance among humanistic values, heartfelt values and insights, and some technical-scientific practice demands. Conventional science is thought to be value-neutral; Caring Science is value-laden, philosophically grounded in values of relationship, context, meaning, and subjective views of reality—acknowledging, but not limited to, empirical-objective physical phenomena alone. Indeed, as Parker Palmer (1987:20) explained, it is "in our modes of knowing that we shape souls by the shape of our knowledge." A renowned educator and transformer of educative minds, Palmer also pointed out that "epistemology is ethic." Knowledge carries ethical, moral shapes that inform and guide our actions; our ways of knowing inform or deform the human soul, according to Palmer.

However, the critique and use of a conventional, objectivist method of knowing and problem solving do not necessarily preclude other domains of knowledge. They are integrated into a new whole, resulting in what draws upon *noetic* knowledge. This evolved approach could be considered *Caritas* Praxis, practice informed by all ways of knowing, being, doing; informed by one's values, ethics, theories, clinical judgment, moral ideals, and so on, as part of the complex dynamics of human relationships and decision making in critical life events and circumstances.

A *Caritas Process* within an expanded model of science, as discussed, critiques limited views of knowledge and asks new ontological, moral, and epistemological questions as to what counts as knowledge. *Caritas Consciousness and Practices* allow for a *noetic** context for science, one not limited to conventional scientific physical phenomena alone (Watson 2002a).

---

* *Noetic* comes from the Greek *nous,* which refers to mind or direct ways of knowing. *Noetic* sciences seek to further explore conventional science in aspects of reality such as mind, consciousness, intentionality, and even spirit, which includes aspects of reality that transcend physical phenomena (Harman 1998; Schlitz, Taylor, and Lewis 1998; Harman 1998; Watson 2002a). Thus, a *noetic science* context would consider Caring/*Caritas* and the subjective-intersubjective world of inner experiences to be legitimate, especially with respect to moral and ontological inquiry.

A Caring Science context for knowledge, evidence, the nursing process, creative problem solving, and decision making reminds us that while nursing needs theory and scientific methodology to guide it in research and practice, it will never be an absolute, pure science such as physics (even though new physics has changed traditional views of hard science). *Caritas Processes* within Caring Science allow for a philosophical-ethical critique of knowledge.

However, for nursing to be a science of caring within a broad ethical and philosophical context, it must work within an established scientific method but be knowledgeable about and open to other ways and to contemporary changes in science and methods generally. The use of scientific problem solving remains the structure for the nursing process but goes beyond a limited interpretation of knowledge and method, honoring unknown subjective phenomena, theories, and conceptual problems as well as scientific data.

DOCUMENTATION OF CARING

As this work evolves, there is a need not only to honor an evolving model of science and problem solving but also to develop approaches to documentation of caring. This issue has recently been addressed by the Resurrection Health System in Chicago. This health care facility, under the leadership of Dr. Linda Ryan (2005) and Susan Rosenberg (2006), has taken steps to develop a new context for charting with an extensive clinical documentation systems upgrade, leading to a new diagnostic category accepted by the North American Nursing Diagnosis Association (NANDA).

The healthcare facility described in the article is part of an eight-hospital organization that adopted Watson's Theory of Caring as part of their nursing philosophy. According to Watson, this theory is an attempt to find and deepen the language specific to nurse caring relations and its many meanings. Yet during the implementation of the theory within the setting described, it was noted that there was no mechanism in the current documentation system for clinical nursing staff to document the patient experience using any language specific to the theory. Nursing members recognized an opportunity to develop a new context in charting during an extensive clinical documentation system upgrade. A discussion of the steps taken and the results within the clinical documentation system supporting the newly adopted caring philosophy are summarized here.

UTILIZING THE LANGUAGE OF JEAN WATSON'S CARING THEORY WITHIN A COMPUTERIZED CLINICAL DOCUMENTATION SYSTEM

Susan Rosenberg, RN, MSN

Senior nursing executives in a Chicago-based healthcare system comprising eight hospitals decided that a new standardized nursing philosophy would be adopted for use by all facilities. At one facility, a 434-bed hospital, the nurse executive was encouraged by a doctorally prepared nursing director to consider using nursing theory as a guide to practice. They decided that nursing theory should be part of the nursing philosophy and determined that the organization's mission and core values is congruent with Watson's Theory of Caring. The facility's vice president brought this information to her colleagues, and these nurse executives agreed that Watson's Theory of Caring would be adopted as part of the system-wide nursing philosophy.

According to Watson,[1] this theory is an attempt to find and deepen the language specific to nurse caring relations and its many meanings. Watson[2] further asserts that the 10 carative factors are dimensions that provide a structure and guide to the theory (see Table 1). They can be used as an expressive tool while directing the assessment, interventions, charting, and full engagement of caring human dimensions of nursing practice. Ference[3] described ways in which nursing administrators can adopt nursing science theories, especially caring theories, to provide nursing services within healthcare organizations. She recommended that the application of nursing science theories occur in a mutual process for administration as well as practice. The nursing practice of concern during this documentation system development was the language used to express the patient experience. The North American Nursing Diagnosis Association International (NANDA-I)[4] states that the important judgements nurses make and the language that expresses them are deeply valued. Yet, during the implementation of the theory within the setting, it was discovered that there was no mechanism within the

Table 1. Watson's Carative Factors[1]

1. The formation of a humanistic-altruistic system of values
2. The instillation of faith-hope
3. The cultivation of sensitivity to one's self and to others
4. The development of a helping-trust relationship
5. The promotion and acceptance of the expression of positive and negative feelings
6. The systematic use of the scientific problem-solving method for decision making
7. The promotion of interpersonal teaching-learning
8. The provision for a supportive, protective, and (or) corrective mental, physical, sociocultural, and spiritual environment
9. Assistance with the gratification of human needs
10. The allowance for existential-phenomenological forces

currently used electronic documentation system for clinical nursing staff to document the patient experience using any language specific to this theory. In the disparity between the newly developed nursing philosophy and documentation, nursing members recognized an opportunity to develop a new context in charting during an extensive clinical documentation system upgrade. Presented here are a discussion of the steps taken and the results achieved within the clinical documentation system to support the newly adopted caring philosophy.

Factors that precipitated the change included the adoption of Watson's theory of caring within nursing philosophy and practice, and the decision to install an upgraded version of the clinical documentation system at all of the hospitals in the healthcare system. Limitations of the current computerized documentation system were that it did not contain the language required to represent the patient experience within the context of the new philosophy and practice, and only 16 characters were allowed for each item documented. Therefore, nursing leaders set out to enhance the system during the upgrade by incorporating the ability to document using language within the context of Watson's Theory of Caring (Figures 1 and 2).

For the new philosophy to become part of nurses' daily practice, leaders of the healthcare facility recognized the need for education regarding the theory. Nursing staff also needed opportunities to participate in this growing process. A group of staff nurses, managers, and other leaders from the facility, known as "The Caring Advocates," was developed to assist in the education and implementation of the theory throughout various clinical settings. Information from the group was shared at unit meetings. Staff were also given the opportunity to communicate theory-related unit endeavors at nursing quality council meetings. Both of these events reinforced education about and adoption of the theory.

One other opportunity taken was to present a lecture by Jean Watson during Nurse's Week 2004. Nurses from the facility as well as throughout the system attended. Nursing leaders from the clinical documentation group, which included members from all hospitals in the system, and selected information service professionals were also invited, because knowledge about the theory would assist in system implementation.

At this lecture, Watson[5] discussed hospitalization as an event that can lead to the loss of human dignity, and stated that it is the nurses' duty to help maintain and restore that dignity. She also described many of the interventions nursing staff can make use of to promote the caring environment. This lecture, along with a review of Jean Watson's other works, provided the support required to build the framework that transformed the current documentation system from a purely technical basis to a system that incorporated information about caring.

During development, the clinical documentation team recognized the required use of a standardized language. According to Werley et al,[6] the Nursing Minimum Data Set (NMDS) was designed to facilitate the abstraction of the minimum, common core of data to describe nursing practice. The nursing care elements of the NMDS include: (1) nursing diagnosis, (2) nursing intervention, (3) nursing outcome, and (4) intensity of nursing service. It was decided that these elements would be considered part of the framework for development of the new caring documentation system.

Review of current literature demonstrated disparity between the ability of the nursing standardized languages, specifically (1) NANDA, (2) Nursing Interventions Classification (NIC), and (3) Nursing Outcomes Classification (NOC), to document the humanistic elements

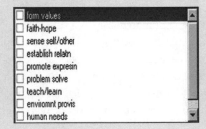

Figure 1. Staff uses scroll bar to access last item "allow forces."

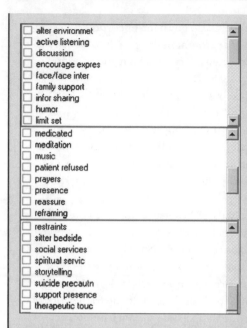

Figure 2. Screen shot of interventions.

within the patient experience. Baumann[7] discusses the text of nursing notes and their relationship to the patient experience as more than an account of vital signs, weight, height, pain assessment, sleep, and output. He further asserts that these notes should reflect the story where there is a character, another person who in a knowledgeable and understandingly present way was with the patient—in short, a nurse. Brown and Crawford8 identified difficulties using NANDA as interaction with patients and stated that nursing diagnosis can never be value-free. They further state that although classification systems may advance professional nursing practice, they may not assist in documenting all the sociological aspects of care.

Aware of the issues regarding the theory and limitations of standardized languages, nursing members began the process of developing new terminology for the documentation system, including a new nursing diagnosis. The diagnosis, as guided by Watson's Theory of Caring, was constructed to assist clinicians in accurately documenting a specific problem, compromised human dignity. It is determined by the patient experience and resulting affects of hospitalization and healthcare promotion modalities. Watson's[1] nursing theory of caring insists that maintaining human dignity is a vital nursing duty and function. As nursing practice is based on nursing theory, appropriate means to communicate this particular patient experience is needed. Walsh and Kowanko[9] assert that nurses have a commitment to the maintenance of patient dignity and that the lack of dignity may lead to poorer health outcomes. Mairis[10] describes the effects of loss of dignity as feelings of ridicule, embarrassment, shame, humiliation, foolishness, degradation, and overt or covert distress. Also stated is that dignity can be affected by a hierarchy in relationships and that hospitals are particularly rich in hierarchies. This hierarchy is illustrated in the perceived relationships as nurses working under the direction of physicians. Soderberg et al[11] suggest that nurse professionals develop qualities to maintain or restore human dignity. They further demonstrate that supporting dignity not only benefits the patient, but the quality of the nurse's work life. The nursing diagnosis label developed for use in this clinical documentation system was Compromised Human Dignity and was submitted to NANDA-I. This diagnosis has been initially accepted by NANDA-I and will be presented at the NANDA-I, NIC, and NOC Conference in March 2006.

Review of interventions as well as outcomes within the system in use demonstrated that it lacked a language that would capture the patient or family experience within the framework of Watson's Theory of Caring. Because the vendor is at the time of writing developing new software and its enhancements will include NANDA, NIC, NOC, and links among them, these existing classifications were reviewed. According to the Center for Nursing Classification and Clinical Effectiveness,[12] NIC is a comprehensive, research-based, standardized classification of interventions that nurses perform. The Center for Nursing Classification and Clinical Effectiveness[13] also defines an intervention as any treatment, based upon clinical judgment and knowledge that a nurse performs to enhance patient/client outcomes. Although use of these languages was considered for this project, the decision was to wait for vendor software upgrades that incorporate the desired languages.

A list of interventions was then developed using Watson's Theory of Caring and was added to those used in the current documentation system. Because the system limited the text of each carative factor to 16 characters, abbreviated legends were constructed (see Tables 1 and 2). The education plans included using a handout containing a list of the carative factors in full text along with its associated abbreviation within the documentation system. A short discussion of each factor with application and example for the clinical setting was developed. Other interventions that demonstrate the caring theory were added. These include reframing, active listening, presence, discussion, and face-to-face interview.

Essential to the documentation process was the inclusion of out-comes. Because NOC will be used in the future when vendor development is completed, reviews of various outcomes and their application were completed using this taxonomy as a reference. The group developed outcome legends that were added to the currently available list, again limited to 16 characters, including (1) decision-making, (2) well-being, (3) spirit well-being, and (4) coping. All of the outcomes developed can be associated with the following indicators as selected by the clinician as (1) improved, (2) deteriorated, and (3) unchanged. These outcome indicators are different from the NOC scales as they do not provide a method of quantifying the outcome. The addition of these outcomes completed the necessary documentation for charting the patient experience as determined within the context of the new nursing philosophy.

Training on the new system included not only the processes to input and change information, but also the new content, including terms associated with Watson's theory. As only 3 hours were given to teach the new system, only 15 minutes were allotted for discussion and demonstration of the theory items. Nurses expressed excitement that the theory was now part of the documentation system. Handbooks were also supplied for nursing units that described how to use the theory for daily documentation of the patient experience. The new system included a query product that allowed extraction of information regarding documentation habits from the system. This product was used to determine if nursing staff were actually using the new theory documentation items. One random search of inpatient records determined that of 274 inpatient documents, 35% had the new label selected and 87% had at least one carative factor documented.

Table 2. Abbreviations of Watson's Carative Factors[1]

1. Form values
2. Faith-hope
3. Sense self/others
4. Establish relation
5. Promote expression
6. Problem solve
7. Teach/learn
8. Environment provis
9. Human needs
10. Allowance forces

Although many organizations incorporate nursing science theory within their nursing philosophies, nurse administrators must ensure that tools are available for nursing staff to document the theory in daily practice. Reviewing current documentation systems and improving them to incorporate standardized terminology assist the expression of the patient experience in the context of the applied theory. When terminology does not exist within current taxonomies to document this experience, nurse leaders then should take an active role in developing and supporting new terminology, as it is needed. As stated by Clark and Lang,[14] "If we cannot name it, we cannot control it, finance it, teach it, research it, or put it into public policy." Further development is now required within current taxonomies to provide NIC and NOC defined as human dignity as this will allow nurses to fully document the patient experience. When nursing interventions are developed using Watson's Theory of Caring,[1] intensity of service could include the 10 carative factors, thereby completing the elements of the NMDS within the con text of this theory. Including intensity of service will assist professional nursing in quantitatively defining practice. Finally, as nursing pursues better definition and development of the terminology required to document the events of the patient experience within the context of a specific theory such as Watson's Theory of Caring, mutuality between nursing theory and nursing practice will be supported.

REFERENCES

1. Watson J. Applying the art and science of human caring. New York, NY: *NLN Publications;* 1994.

2. Watson J. *Nursing and the Philosophy and Science of Caring.* Niwot, CO: University of Colorado Press; 1995.

3. Ference HM. Nursing science theories and administration. In: Henry B., Arndt C., Divonconti M.,Mainer-Tomey A., eds. *Dimensions of Nursing Administration, Theory, Research, Education, and Practice.* Boston, Mass: Blackwell Scientific; 1989:121–131.

4. NANDA-I Membership Information. Available at: http://www.nanda.org/html/member_brochure.htm. Accessed January 29, 2004.

5. Watson J. *Living Caring Theory.* Lecture at Resurrection Medical Center, Chicago, IL. May 7, 2004.

6. Werley H, Ryan P, Zorn C. The nursing minimum data set (NMDS): a frame work for the organization of nursing language. In: American Nurses Association Steering Committee on Databases to Support Clinical Nursing

Practice, ed. *Nursing Data Systems: The Emerging Framework.* Washington, DC: American Nurses Publishing; 1995:19–30.

7. Baumann S. Nurses notes: the text of nursing. *Nurs Sci Q.* 2004; 17(3):267.

8. Brown B, Crawford P. Putting the debate on nursing language in context. *Nurs Stand.* 1999;14(1):41–43.

9. Walsh K, Kowanko I. Nurses' and patients' perceptions of dignity. *Int J Nurs Pract.* June 2002;8(3):143–151.

10. Mairis E. Concept clarification of professional practice—dignity. *J Adv Nurs.* May 1994;19(5):947–953.

11. Soderberg A, Gilje F, Norberg A. Dignity in situations of ethical difficulty in intensive care. *Intensive Crit Care Nurs.* June 1997;13(3):135–144.

12. University of Iowa, College of Nursing. Nursing intervention classification overview. Available at: http://www.nursing.uiowa.edu/centers/cncce/nic/nicoverview.htm. Accessed January 29, 2004.

13. University of Iowa, College of Nursing. Nursing outcome classification overview. http://www.nursing.uiowa.edu/centers/cncce/noc/nocoverview.htm. Accessed January 29, 2004.

14. Clark J, Lang NM. Nursing's next advance: an international classification for nursing practice. *Int Nurs Rev.* 1992; 39:109–111, 128.

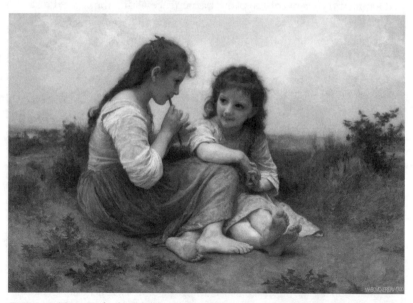

Figure 12. Two Girls, *by Adolphe William Bouguereau. Collection, The Denver Art Museum.*

CHAPTER ELEVEN

From **CARATIVE FACTOR 7:** *Promotion of*
Interpersonal Teaching and Learning
to **CARITAS PROCESS 7:** *Engage in Genuine Teaching-Learning*
Experience That Attends to Unity of Being and Subjective Meaning—
Attempting to Stay Within the Other's Frame of Reference

Nurses have long been clear about a teaching role, even though it often does not receive attention or systematic follow-through. Moreover, the intersubjective, relational aspect of the process is often not made explicit. For example, even though teaching and the imparting of health information, self-caring approaches, and so forth are mainstream, the dialectic, transpersonal aspects of teaching-learning and the importance of the caring relationship as context are often overlooked.

Learning is more than receiving information, facts, or data. It involves a meaningful, trusting relationship that is intersubjective; the nature of the relationship as well as the form and context of teaching affects the process. There is an honoring of the whole person. The content as well as the readiness of the patient to receive the information are critical variables. The meaning the content has for the person—intellectually, symbolically, and culturally as well as literally—

affects his or her ability to receive and process the information. The process of genuine teaching becomes transpersonal, in that the experience, the relationship, and the meaning and significance of the experience affect both parties within the teaching encounter. Thus, the relationship lives on beyond the context of the teaching, informing the life and behavior and actions that flow from the experience.

Dated words such as "compliance" were used in relation to a person following through on information and advice. The *Caritas Model* of teaching-learning does not operate on the concept of "compliance," in that an authentic relational model and process is not one of authority and use of a professional, superior position with an authoritarian approach of control and power over another, with information given out and expectations to comply with that information. Rather, the *Caritas Process* of teaching-learning is more relational, trusting, exploratory, engaging, and ultimately liberating for patient and others. It involves power and control with, not over, the learner. Teaching-learning in the practice of *Caritas* results in self-knowledge, self-care, self-control, and even self-healing possibilities. There is a mutuality whereby the *Caritas Nurse* helps the other generate his or her own problem solving, decisions, constructive solutions, and actions that are able to best serve him or her.

A *Caritas* teaching-learning process depends upon the nurse's ability to accurately detect another's feelings, thoughts, readiness, mood, and so on, and then to connect with and access the other's perceptions, feelings, concerns, knowledge, and understandings. The Caring process requires openness to the other's feelings, knowledge, information, and level of intellectual understandings, as well as openness and readiness for learning.

One of the core skills in this process is being able to genuinely access, stay within, and work from the other person's frame of reference rather than from one's own reference point. The teaching-learning process thus requires a meaningful relationship as well as timing and sensitivity to the teaching moment. It is creative as well as purposive; it requires conscious planning and knowledgeable, informed action.

While the traditional nursing educational-teaching role was one of imparting information, this was usually done in conventional ways and around conventional issues, such as diabetes education, birthing classes, medication administration, and so on. The *Caritas* transpersonal teaching process is more personalized, relational, and meaningful, consistent with the individual's specific condition, needs, readiness, and so on.

However, an even more extensive approach that represents the next evolution involves still another level of depth with respect to *Caritas Nursing*. This is the shift toward Health-Wellness-Healing Coaching— what I call *Caritas Coaching*, which embraces transpersonal and unity views of teaching but goes into greater depth in working within the other's frame of reference.

This coaching requires a more advanced approach to teaching-learning; it requires more specific skills with respect to caring relationships as well as ways to actually assist another in finding his or her best solutions, options, and strategies to address and solve self-identified issues and needs. The plan for coaching is based on the other's inner goals and self-defined, self-motivated pursuits. It involves affirming, encouraging, following up, and celebrating with another's successes. It invites personal growth and maturing, helping the other discover his or her support systems, the environment that reinforces the individual's goals; *Caritas Coaching* helps another face his or her shadow side of negative habits and ways of thinking and find inner strengths and gifts. Through this expanded model, the nurse becomes more of a sojourner along with the other, helping the other find new energy, time, and ways to excel by working from the inside out, connecting with his or her inner spirit and authentic longings for self.

In other words, in *Caritas Coaching* the person becomes his or her own best problem solver; the individual is his or her own best source for finding unique creative solutions for meeting goals and a vision for change. Thus, *Caritas Coaching* is a very different model than conventional teaching-learning approaches whereby the one with authority and knowledge imparts information and content to another—often with no comprehension of the context, meaning, and relationship with respect to the other's inner strivings, hopes, deep longings, and needs. The *Caritas Coach* continues to be a resource to the person even after the person has met his or her goals or had a setback.

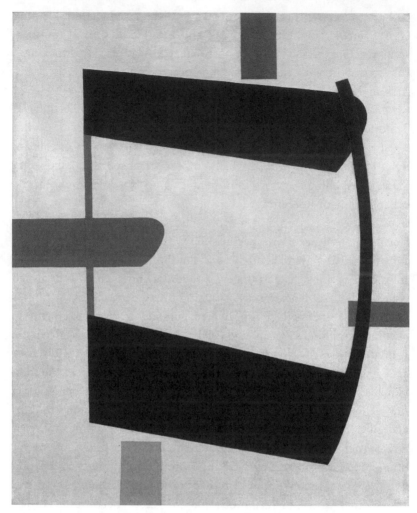

Figure 13. Equilibre, *by Jean Hélion. Collection, The Denver Art Museum.*

CHAPTER TWELVE

From **CARATIVE FACTOR 8:** *Attending to a Supportive,*
Protective, and/or Corrective Mental, Physical,
Societal, and Spiritual Environment
to **CARITAS PROCESS 8:** *Creating a Healing Environment*
at All Levels

COMFORT

Comfort measures can be supportive, protective, and even corrective of a person's inner and outer environments. The environment of hospitals, while dramatically improved over the past two decades, is still too inflexible and bound by tradition, controls, schedules, and routines to meet the individual needs of patients and family members.

Some of the comfort measures identified in my original text still hold today as basic guidelines (Watson 1979). These and other approaches continue to serve only as examples but are consistent with Nightingale's views that still need attention (Watson 1979:90).

- Remove noxious stimuli from the external environment (bright lights, loud and sudden noises, inadequate heating, poor ventilation, untidy surroundings, and so on).

- Give attention to the patient's position and frequently change that position.

- Make the bed safe, comfortable, clean, and attractive (see the "Zen of Bed-Making" in Watson 1999:237–240).

- Relieve muscle or emotional tension with massage, breath work, range-of-motion exercise, back rub, therapeutic touch, use of music, sound, visualization-relaxation approaches, use of aroma-therapy, other nursing arts, energy therapies.

- Perform therapeutic nursing procedures (apply warm moist packs, warm bath, administer prescribed pain-relieving medications with affirmative statements, inhalation exercises, provide helpful information, and so on).

- Identify the implications and meaning of the illness and condition for the patient, and draw upon multiple available, creative resources for support, protection; prepare patient for what to anticipate; increase self-control, self-caring, self-knowledge, and self-generating responses for choices, alternatives.

- Engage in combination of any and all Carative Factors/*Caritas Processes* to best meet the patient's needs for a healing environment and comfort, drawing upon multiple creative ways of problem solving congruent with patient's needs and professional caring practices.

In addition to these specific examples, the *Caritas Nurse* can utilize numerous other techniques: sitting with patient and family members, rearranging the patient's room, placing the bed properly, providing a view of nature, closing or opening the window, listening to patient, contacting family members, and so on. Nightingale identified these methods and more in her timeless treatise on nursing (1969).

Another deeper level of considering comfort involves controlling pain and human suffering, which are very subjective and affected by the patient's experience, belief system, and the meaning of the pain—including spiritual and cultural meanings and associations with respect to pain and suffering generally. This focus of concern is a separate area that requires full-time attention.

For our purposes here, it is important to emphasize that the nurse's appreciation of, respect for, and acknowledgment of the spiritual and cultural significance of pain and suffering in a person's life (regardless of one's culture-belief system) are a form of comfort in their own right. Nurses have an opportunity as well as an obligation to become familiar with the spiritual, cultural, and religious meanings associated with pain, comfort, and caring. Thus, in this *Caritas Process,* the nurse can be a lifeline between the often impersonal "case" environmental responses and the patient's subjective cultural and spiritual needs and beliefs that are honored as part of the provision of a healing environment at all levels—seeing and honoring the "face" of the other and his or her personal, individual needs.

SAFETY

The original focus of this Carative Factor remains the same, even as it has evolved and continues to evolve. Indeed, issues related to safety, such as falls, injuries, infections, skin care, sterilization, hand washing, over- or under-medication, all types of medication errors—wrong person, wrong medication, wrong method of administration, and so on—along with other issues, such as safety of medical devices, bathing-toilet access and equipment, restraining devices, radiation contamination, pollution-toxicity levels, and others, have been the subject of national news exposés as well as scientific Institute of Medicine studies, reports, warnings, and attention. Safety is a basic component of professional nursing and *Caritas Processes.* Safety concerns affect all of the nurse's activities related to supporting, protecting, and correcting the environment for healing at all levels.

To feel safe and protected is a basic need. To experience the absence of threats or danger in the environment is critical to a person's well-being. It is the nurse's ethical obligation to ensure safety. Environmental issues are presenting concerns for both nurse and patient.

The nurse's concern for safety and well-being includes an appreciation of the various developmental and emotional factors that contribute to a person's belief that the environment is safe or unsafe. Depending upon his or her background and trust in the current situation, the patient behaves in a variety of ways to create a sense of safety and self-control over the environment. The *Caritas Nurse* demonstrates concern for safety at multiple levels, including knowledge of, appreciation for, and tolerance of behaviors—even idiosyncratic behaviors—that contribute to a person's sense of well-being and safety.

With regard to attending to safety issues, the *Caritas Nurse* makes sure to address the person by his or her preferred name and to make direct eye contact when appropriate. The *Caritas Nurse* uses a technical occasion as a caring occasion, allowing a caring moment to emerge from the presenting situation. For example, in instances where medication administration is using bar codes to ensure safety rather than "work around" the bar code system, the nurse can use the occasion to correctly identify the person, to connect with the patient at the human level. Thus, the *Caritas Nurse* can use the moment as an occasion to touch the other while swiping the bar code, turning a routine requirement into a caring occasion and a potential caring moment. Likewise, when administering medications, the *Caritas Nurse* pauses and "centers"/empties out so she or he can focus and more clearly concentrate on administering the correct medication to the correct patient with the correct dosage and the correct route at the designated time.

Accidents remain a leading cause of death among persons in all age groups. Maintaining safety is especially crucial for those who are very ill, confused, anxious, overly excited, or experiencing apprehension over a loss of control in their environment. Conditions such as weakness, sensory deprivation, sensory overload, incapacitation, disorientation, someone heavily medicated, organic brain damage, senility, and so on, make patients highly vulnerable. These conditions and more require the nurse to take extra care to ensure that the person's environment is supportive, corrective, and protective. Patients whose physical and mental conditions are compromised usually need help from the nurse to modify their usual responses to facilitate self-control over their functions, and the nurse can help provide measures to address the patients' lack of control, to meet their needs more authentically and safely. Safety considerations in the environment are critical needs largely confined to the professional nurse's domain of assessment and intervention. This Carative Factor acknowledges the nurse's special and unique role in providing for a safe, supportive, protective, and/or corrective environment for patients at all levels and all ages.

PRIVACY

Privacy is a major factor to consider with this Carative Factor. The depersonalization and intimate questions, procedures, and treatments connected with hospitalization contribute to the patient's privacy concerns. Hospital personnel's expectation that the patient will share intimate information and expose his or her body without reserve also contributes to the patient's loss of privacy. Often the basic support, protection, or correction the nurse provides in the patient's environment is intended to preserve the patient's privacy.

Privacy was linked to health in the early work of Maslow (1968), in that healthy people have a strong need for privacy. Some privacy concerns include:

- The right to exclude others from certain knowledge about oneself
- The awareness and appreciation that others have the same privileges one desires for oneself
- Factors of time, place, manner, and amount of information
- Attempts to exclude oneself from others that may be voluntary and temporary and that may involve physical and/or psychological exclusion.

Privacy often maintains the patient's human dignity and integrity. A violation of privacy is often a violation of a person's dignity. Humiliation, embarrassment, and depersonalization often result from an invasion of privacy.

One of the explicit dimensions of human caring theory and the *Caritas Model* is the preservation of human dignity. However, this feature has not always been made explicit in nursing practice until very recently. For example, the North American Nursing Diagnosis Association (NANDA) recently reviewed inclusion of a new/revised diagnosis, "Compromised Human Dignity," which indicated that people are at risk for loss of respect and honor (Rosenberg 2006).

HUMAN DIGNITY

Some of the identified risk factors with this new NANDA diagnosis include (Rosenberg 2006):

- Exposure of one's body
- Perceived invasion of privacy
- Inadequate participation in decision making
- Disclosure of confidential information
- Loss of control of body functions
- Use of undefined medical terms
- Perceived dehumanizing treatment
- Perceived humiliation
- Stigmatizing labels.

It is a breakthrough that these threats to privacy are now being named and identified as specific acts that need caring attention to alleviate.

Privacy needs and human dignity overlap in that attending to these needs is a very important function for human behavior and preserving the unique humanness and integrity of self and other. Steps in attending to these needs include, for example:

- Maintaining personal autonomy, one's uniqueness as a human being.

- Providing emotional release and a sense of safety and protection from stress and strains in the outer-world environment.

- Engaging in self-affirmation, reflection, by which one is able to pause, reflect, explore, and integrate feelings and experiences. This function of preserving privacy and sustaining human dignity may be closely related to the spiritual or creative-meditative activities that bring meaning to one's life.

- Allowing for limited and protective, intimate communication. This function of privacy and human dignity allows for safely sharing confidential, intimate information and setting boundaries and social distances in trusting interpersonal/transpersonal relationships.

Obviously, a number of variables affect privacy and the ways it manifests itself in social-cultural behavior and helps sustain human dignity. For example, some African tribes have no word or equivalent term for privacy. Westerners have attempted to explain the concept of privacy to people in those tribes, but the concept closest to it is that of the hermit, a private person who does not like other people or civilizations. In other words, in some cultures the concept of privacy as we know it in the Western world does not exist. Other cultures often have a conflict with privacy notions, placing communal life and people's unity, sharing, and engaging over individual needs and concerns. Thus, for example, a group social-humanitarian focus takes precedence over individualism. The People's Republic of China, some societies in the South Pacific islands, and others are examples of such cultures.

The concept of preserving human dignity is universal, however. Indeed, one basic right of human dignity includes privacy. The *Caritas Nurse* recognizes these basic rights for others as well as for self. Professional integrity, dignity, and confidentiality are integral aspects of privacy. A caring-trusting relationship is often dependent on this aspect of maintaining human dignity.

Supporting a person's right to privacy can often instill faith and hope, helping to sustain a caring-trusting relationship. Privacy is a basic component of this Carative Factor and expands the attention the nurse brings to the individual needs of others as he or she seeks to preserve human dignity and the integrity of self and others.

CLEAN AESTHETIC SURROUNDINGS
Clean aesthetic surroundings are a basic element of this Carative Factor. The testimony of nursing across time, from Florence Nightingale forward, highlights the importance of clean surroundings. For this reason, cleanliness is often associated with patient care. However, in the past, custodial institutional care was sterile and industrial, depersonalizing and drab. Such institutional darkness that is faceless, harsh, and sterile can make us feel unwell, exhausted, and disconnected from our self and our source of energy (Watson 1999). Such anonymity of our environment can be "life sapping"; consider that historically, hospitals were considered "warehouses for bodies" instead of places for the soul (Watson 1999:243). Such separation evokes the feeling that "you know no one and no one knows you" as a person, and no one cares.

However, even at a superficial level, Nightingale integrated noise, sound, light, air, taste, sanitation, water, cleanliness, aesthetic beauty, variety, views, pets, trees, nature, children, music, color, form, flowers, paintings, proper nutrition, a comfortable bed, and sleep as natural environmental modalities that promoted healing (Watson 1999:253). Recent developments in hospital architecture and design are introducing elements of beauty, local color, decoration, and historical references, thereby helping to reintroduce harmonious connections, wholeness, and relationships between and among people and their environments.

A personalized, pleasant, aesthetic environment elevates one's experience. There is often a need for order, beauty, and symmetry as a means of connecting with the human soul; such order and equilibrium can help bring closure and completion to an experience, give ritual and meaning to an important event. Nightingale was clear that beauty is healing; the need to beautify one's surroundings, and doing so, make a person feel better about self and other. Such efforts introduce these aesthetic dimensions as expressions of humanity and a way to preserve human and humane connections. Indeed, environments that contain unpleasant odors, medicinal smells, and other noxious stimuli produce negative emotions and increase heart rate and anxiety, whereas pleasant aromas, color, and pleasing sensory elements lower people's blood pressure and heart rate (Malkin 1992:20).

Today, progressive healing therapies seek to unify nature and health. These therapies include the intentional use of clean aesthetic surroundings, organic shapes, color, texture, and lighting, as well as modalities such as mineral baths, massage, music, sculpture, painting, art therapy, and all kinds of expressive arts, to harmonize the human-environment-natural surroundings, allowing beauty and aesthetics into the caring-healing process.

While acknowledging and building upon the original text of Carative Factor 8 (incorporating the well-known aspects of safety, privacy, comfort, clean aesthetic surroundings, and so on), it is also important to bring human-environmental-nature-field consciousness to another level as part of my evolved turn toward *Caritas Process* 8.

In *Caritas Process* 8, in which we create a healing environment at all levels—physical environment as well as the nonphysical, subtle environment of energy and consciousness—wholeness, beauty, safety, comfort, dignity, and peace are potentiated. In this expanded process, environment takes on an entirely new meaning whereby the nurse is *in* the environment, addressing all the above aspects of environment, but in the *Caritas Process* the nurse *becomes* or *is* the environment (Quinn 1992).

Nightingale considered environment core to a nursing paradigm. As part of an evolved approach to environment, the original goal for this Carative Factor, consistent with Nightingale, was to strengthen comfort, privacy, safety, aesthetics, and so forth, resulting in supporting the patient's well-being through holistic attention to the physical, mental, sociocultural, and spiritual aspects of the health-healing environment.

In the *Caritas Nursing* model, the concept and notion of environment undergo a reconceptualization, resulting in a transformation. While still attending to conventional physical-environmental concerns and issues, nonphysical concepts now come to our attention: for example, concepts such as consciousness, intentionality, energy, and awareness of the *Nurse-self* come into focus. New questions emerge as to the nature of the subtle environment as well as the more obvious physical environment. These expanded and transformative views of environment represent my evolved thinking and are enhanced by the framework proposed by Quinn (1992).

EXPANDED LEVELS OF ENVIRONMENTAL CONCEPTUALIZATION
This expanded view of the *Caritas* environment moves

- From an exclusive, external physical-environmental focus (whereby the nurse alters, controls, and influences the physical surroundings in specific ways—consistent with original Carative Factor)
- Toward considering notions such as "environmental field" and "re-patterning-the-field" for patient healing (whereby the nurse and patient are integral to the broader field—consistent with caring modalities in Watson 1999) (Quinn 1992)
- To a consideration of the *"Nurse-as-the Environment"* (Quinn 1992).

Quinn's (1992) work is helpful in seeking to clarify my evolutionary thinking and the transition from conventional views of environment toward a transformative *Caritas* view. For example, in her classic work (1992), Quinn identified several ways of examining environment within nursing practice:

- First, by acknowledging that both the nurse and the patient are in the physical environment, both looking out into a shared physical space. The nurse in this framework attends to the most basic essentials of environment, such as privacy, comfort, lighting, safety, cleanliness, aesthetics, and so forth, including acknowledging spiritual needs. These are foundationally important aspects of the caring process in nursing and one of the core Carative Factors.

- Second, however, we go beyond the basic Carative essentials as we expand our disciplinary and theory-guided practice. Now we are invited to consider environment at a theory-guided practice level. Were we to consider Rogers's (1970, 1994) view of the human-environmental field and an expanded view of nurse and patient as integral within the environment, affecting the entire field, we then must rethink environment and the nurse's role and place in the space.

- This second evolved view builds on the first, but in addition to considering the nurse and patient as sharing the physical space and the nurse as altering that space to meet the patient's basic needs, the nurse now has to consider *self* as part of the environmental field. This view introduces concepts such as patterning/ re-patterning of the environment to promote healing and deeper caring.

- Furthermore, in considering environmental field at this deeper level, the nurse working within a holistic caring consciousness would consider introducing caring-healing modalities, such as music, intentional touch, sound, art, aromatherapy, visualization, relaxation, and other nursing arts, as well as healing arts approaches to enhance healing and help the patient "be-in-right-relation" (Quinn personal communication, 1986).

- While Quinn did not necessarily locate her ideas within a Caring Science context, as I do here, she nevertheless invited a third level of consideration of environment. This third view is consistent with Caring Science and the *Caritas Nursing* consciousness proposed throughout this text. This deeper conceptualization of environment takes into consideration the subtle environment and both the nonphysical and physical surroundings. The notion of "environmental field" incorporates the more subtle energetic nature of environment, as it must—for example, the presence, consciousness, and intentionality of caring-healing practitioners.

- This third level of (*Caritas*) consciousness-environment invites us to reconsider our understanding of the *Practitioner-Self*, no longer separate from the patient's environment but integral to the patient's field. Thus, we have an obligation to pay attention to the presence, consciousness, and intentionality of the *nurse-self* as an energetic, vibrational field, integral to and one with the patient's field, thus affecting the whole.

As we move to these evolved perspectives on environment, environmental field, and so on, new questions can be asked (Quinn 1992; Watson 2005:94–95):

- If I *Am the Environment*, how can I *Be* a more caring-healing environment?
- How can I become a safe, healing space for this person? To draw out healing, wholeness?
- How can my heart-centered (*Caritas*) presence and loving-caring consciousness help align in this moment with the spirit of this person?
- How can I use my consciousness, my intentionality, my *Being*, my presence, my voice, touch, face, heart, hands, and so on, for healing?

The nurse becomes more attuned to the fact that his or her mood, demeanor, and presence affect the human-environmental field, for better or for worse. The caring relationship and environment are generated by the nurse's heartfelt, loving presence and the consciousness he or she holds, helping to shape the patient's health and healing experience as well as the nurse's own experiences.

WHAT WE HOLD IN OUR HEART MATTERS IN CREATING A *CARITAS* ENVIRONMENT

This heartfelt *Caritas* thinking is based on the given that we are interconnected with all of life through the universal field of infinite Love

(Levinas 1969). Intentional touch and energetic caring modalities are examples of how one works within the unified field to repattern in the direction of expanded consciousness. Quinn goes further by using the metaphor of sound, suggesting that the pattern and vibration of the nurse's higher energetic field of (*Caritas*) consciousness become a tuning fork, resonating at a healing (Love) vibratory frequency in which the patient attunes to or resonates with that (higher) frequency. In this expanded *Caritas* view, we acknowledge that *what the nurse holds in her or his heart matters* (M. Smith personal communication, 2007). The heart sends messages to the mind, radiating energetically into the field and guiding actions, opening a new field of possibilities in the moment.

This line of thinking is consistent with the human caring theoretical notion that caring consciousness transcends time, space, and physicality and is dominant over the physical (Watson 1999). This (*Caritas*) awareness alters the human-environmental field and helps the patient access his or her inner healer (or helps the other to be in "right-relation"); thus, such an environmental presence can at least potentiate an inner healing processes.

In other words, holding authentic, heartfelt, positive thoughts such as loving-kindness, caring, healing, forgiveness, and so forth, vibrates at a higher level than having lower thoughts, such as competition, fear, greed, anxiety, hostility, and similar thoughts (Watson 1999). If one holds higher-thought consciousness, the entire field can be, and is being, repatterned by the nurse's consciousness. The nurse-self, the *Caritas Nurse,* then indeed *Becomes* the environment, affecting the entire field. A caring moment is more likely to manifest in the "now," informed by the higher consciousness being communicated by the nurse's (*Caritas*) consciousness.

CARITAS ENVIRONMENTAL FIELD MODEL

In this expanded consciousness view of environment, we evolve in our theories and in our science; we are called to look again at how we knowingly participate/co-participate in our unitary field. In the *Caritas* environmental model, we can no longer view the environment or the practitioner as "out there," separate and distinct from us as a "case" disconnected from the wider, deeper unitary field to which we all belong. This perspective turns toward the universal Love we call upon in our lives and our work and our world. However, it requires personal-professional awakening and an evolution toward a higher-deeper level of consciousness.

CHAPTER THIRTEEN

From **CARATIVE FACTOR 9:** *Assistance with*
Gratification of Human Needs
to **CARITAS PROCESS 9:** *Administering Sacred Nursing*
Acts of Caring-Healing by Tending to Basic Human Needs

Or do you not know that your body is a temple of the Holy Spirit
within you?

CORINTHIANS I, KING JAMES BIBLE

In a Caring Science model, it is necessary to remind ourselves
that we are spirit made whole; non-manifest to manifest field,
connected to and Belonging to the Infinity of cosmos and the
Universe, before separating as individuals.

WATSON (2005:111)

It seems that somewhere along the way we have forgotten that one
of the greatest honors and privileges one can have as a nurse is to
be able to care for another person. Such personal, intimate connections and relations touch on the Holy, as well as the horrific at
times. Caring (and the need for caring) is such a vulnerable place;
first, because we come face-to-face with our own humanity

143

and ourselves. In this place, we realize that one person's level of humanity reflects back on the other. The other reason this place of caring and healing transcends medical thinking and conventional science is, when we locate ourselves in this new space, we are remembering our own and others' humanity and our shared belonging to the infinity of Universal Field of Infinite Love (Levinas 1969) that embraces Spirit. We are remembering we are touching the life force, the very soul of another person, hence ourselves.

WATSON (2005:61, SLIGHTLY MODIFIED)

One of the privileges of nursing and its role in interacting with humanity is that nurses have access to the human body. Nurses have the intimate honor of helping others gratify their most basic human needs, especially when vulnerable. It seems that somewhere along the way nursing detoured from this connection and forgot that one of the greatest honors one can have is to take care of another person when in need. It is the ultimate contribution to society and to people's human needs—a gift to civilization (Watson 2005).

As nurses begin to work from a *Caritas Consciousness*, they take a sense of sacredness into all aspects of their life and work. It is here that nurses and nursing "manifest at the highest level" (Dossey, Keegan, and Guzzetta 2005:231). This view brings us face-to-face with the mystery and infinity of humanity itself and with all life processes. As we enter this deeper *Caritas* dimension of our life and work and world, we understand more deeply the sacredness of Caring and understand that each act we commit is part of a larger whole.

Martinsen (2006) reminds us of the notion of "dwelling." Nursing has a responsibility to attend to that which is more than the satisfaction of needs and that is related to life-enhancing space, attending to and creating rooms wherein one can find calm, rest, and "dwell." Nursing must do so without robbing the body of calmness and rest, seeking to avoid invading the room with rapidity and busyness so the other loses his or her physical and bodily footing and becomes homeless, so to speak, robbing the body of relations and rhythms (Martinsen 2006:9).

It is the "dwelling" notion (more than just helping to satisfy basic human needs) that takes on a philosophical view of caring that allows one to "see with the heart's eye," "emphasizing the importance of being seen in such a way that one becomes significant to the one who sees" (Martinsen 2006:11).

When considering basic needs and administering *Caritas Nursing* as a sacred act as opposed to a physical task alone, human beings are cared for in a loving, kind way in which they feel secure and safe and protected. The *Caritas Nurse* creates space and places for "dwelling," whereby the "body inhabits the room in a good way . . . the body is able to embrace experiences as [dignifying] life sustaining, in the midst of pain and suffering; letting the human dwell" (Martinsen 2006:16).

This view of "dwelling," from Foucault (1975), addresses the hospital or sickroom, whereby the nurse helps another person move beyond the professional "gaze" (the "case" mentality) to the notion of creating an individual dwelling space for healing. This view is in contrast to architecture and rooms in hospitals that possess "innumerable petty mechanisms, flawless instrumentations to objectify and control the individual's totality, leaving them stripped and naked to the gaze of others [the professionals]" (Foucault quoted in Martinsen 2006:16).

In this model of *Caritas Nursing*, one makes explicit that when touching another person, you are not touching just the body physical but also the embodied spirit. Indeed, when a nurse touches another person, she or he is touching not only the body but also the other's mind, the other's heart, and the other's soul—the other's very life source.

From Nightingale forward, nursing and nursing leaders have long recognized that the physical body is not the "eternal aspect" of human nature but the "vehicle" of the spirit or soul essence of the human person that dwells within the body physical (Macrae 2001). Nevertheless, tending to the body physical has often become the focus of patient care. In this model the care needs and approaches of physical-nonphysical care cannot be separated from the web of other relationships—social, environmental, ecological, systems, spiritual, and otherwise (Jarrin 2006).

My original (1979) work related to this Carative Factor organized basic needs into lower- and higher-order needs, using Maslow's theory as a template. However, this revised version of the book will not order this chapter using that outdated framework. I continue to organize around a framework that integrates conventional basic needs but now within a context of what can be thought of as *Caritas Nursing* art/acts, or, more deeply, sacred arts of nursing. As these acts are identified, we acknowledge that nurses respond to the most primal, instinctual, often embarrassing, private needs of another, touching their whole being with each act. I repeat: it is the "dwelling" notion (more than just helping to satisfy basic human needs) that takes on a philosophical view of caring that allows one to "see with the heart's eye" (Martinsen 2006:11).

Nurses have the honored position of entering another's private physical-environmental surroundings as well as having access to one's sacred body-physical-personal private space. Nurses enter this space when carrying out acts, processes, and functions of caring for another that the person/family often conducts in the privacy and intimacy of their own homes. But when another is vulnerable, injured, incapacitated, ill, weak, frail, suffering, confused, and dependent, *Caritas Nurses*—in a spirit of loving-kindness, with an intentional consciousness of dignity and honoring other, combined with "Caring Literacy," knowledge, and skill—administer to another. As the nurse carries out these basic need functions with a caring-loving consciousness, as perhaps an ultimate gift to this person, she or he is bringing spirit into the physical plane, helping the other have space to "dwell" in his or her body as well as in the institutional environment. This *Caritas Nursing* consciousness makes new connections between basic needs and evolving spiritual needs, intentionally aware that each physical act is touching the spirit of the person and making a difference in that person's life in that moment.

However, any presenting need can be related to self-survival, even if existential-spiritual in nature; our needs are not restricted to the biophysical in the usual sense of "basic needs." These deeper, evolving human needs beyond physical survival encompass the human in a unified way that expands and deepens our evolving humanity and being-in-the-world. Examples of other aspects of human evolution include:

- The need for work-purpose, contributing to something beyond self, something larger than self

- The need for achievement—self-efficacy, self-esteem, self-concept
- The need for affiliation—family, love, and belonging
- The need for knowledge—understanding, making meaning (of life situation)
- The need for beauty-aesthetics
- The need for self-expression, creativity
- The need for play and relaxation
- The need for an evolving self-actualization that is spiritually meaningful
- The need to connect with that which is greater than self—to surrender to a higher source with a sense of awe toward the mystery and wonder of life, whether humanity itself, nature, God, Spirit, or a Divine universe.

Nevertheless, while all these needs are holographic in nature, each one embodies and affects all the others. Without attending to the most basic physical human needs, one's physical survival is vulnerable, preventing deeper evolution. Any basic need on the physical plane can be considered a need of the embodied soul.

In the past, it was generally assumed that a person can take care of, or assist another with, basic physical needs, separate from the whole of his or her humanity and the energetic field of the individual's life force. In this evolved model of *Caritas Consciousness*, we realize that this is not possible. Soul care as well as physical care is required to respond to each and all needs, in that the whole of spirit/soul is in each physical and nonphysical need and is embodied in the physical plane of the body.

When one touches another's body, as mentioned, the individual is touching not only the physical body but also the person's mind, heart, and soul at some level. A *Caritas Nurse* is conscious and aware of this perspective in assisting another with basic needs, at whatever level of need is presenting. The nurse responds to these needs as a privilege, an honor, and a sacred act in assisting this person. The *Caritas Nurse* appreciates that in this one act, he or she is connecting with and contributing both to the spirit of that person and to oneself.

CHAPTER FOURTEEN

Administering Sacred Nursing Acts—Further Development
of CARATIVE FACTOR/CARITAS PROCESS 9

HUMAN NEED FOR FOOD AND FLUID

With the backdrop of the discussion of broader views of human needs, it can now be stated that the human need for food and fluid is both physical and metaphysical; it is more than the need for survival. In all cultures and occasions, eating and food have intrinsic meaning for emotional relationships, communication, and feelings of love, friendship, contentment, comfort, support, social life—good feelings. We do not simply ingest food and fluid; we incorporate the associated sensations, surroundings, the other's human presence, sound, energetic mood, the consciousness, if you will, of the person preparing or offering the food. We take all of this into the body and into our experience of eating and being fed.

This need is very symbolic and full of meaning beyond the physical need for food and drink. This need, with all its real and symbolic and metaphoric meanings, is basic for physical and emotional survival and is considered one of the biophysical needs.

However, rather than develop information about this need, I am going to explore it from the standpoint of nursing assisting another in meeting his or her needs. Associated with this need is the art/act, the sacred act, if you will, of "feeding another human," metaphorically as well as literally. It is associated with knowing how to give and receive from another human. Eating behaviors, habits, associations, food taste, and desires are directly associated with the meanings and relationships of eating, drinking, and symbolic aspects.

I had a dream not long ago in which I witnessed a nurse going into a patient's room, almost throwing a glass of water to the patient in his bed, then turning around and walking away. The nurse thrust the glass into the patient's face, and water spilled all over the patient's bedclothes. The nurse ignored the fact that she had done this and just walked out of the patient's room.

Rather than hand the patient the water in such a way as to ensure that he received it, and rather than help him receive the glass of water or at least assist him after the water had spilled on him, the nurse basically turned her back on the patient and left him wet and uncared for. As I witnessed this in my dream, I was astonished at the nurse's behavior. In the dream I called out to the nurse: "Wait a minute! That is unacceptable; it is not OK, what just happened. There is a way to give something to someone in such a way that they can receive it, in contrast to just throwing something at someone without any consciousness of how to participate, give, and receive with another."

This dream was informative in that we sometimes think caring means letting people get by with uncaring acts, especially in a professional nursing practice, without confronting and acknowledging the destructive behavior. Caring does not mean ignoring careless acts or incompetent behavior. This act in my dream was incompetent as well as cruel. If one cares authentically, it is not acceptable to allow behavior that is inappropriate or destructive to go unchallenged or uncorrected.

The second part of the dream, especially with respect to the way the nurse thrust the water upon the patient, was the other message. The nurse's ignorance, lack of mindful consciousness, lack of skill, lack of *Caritas* awareness, caring incompetence, absence of Caring Literacy, if you will, illiteracy of caring, all contributed to a careless, destructive, and thoughtless act toward another. Offering food or a drink to another, patient or otherwise, is a sacred act; it is a reciprocal act of giving and receiving, helping another meet a most basic nurturing human need—a human need that is basic to the nurse as well as the patient.

In this *Caritas Nursing* Framework, the human need for food and fluid is considered an essential part of human survival. Food / drink is symbolic; it is sacred, in that food comes from the sacred circle of life and sustains the life-energy source for human living, growing, thriving, and evolving. It emphasizes the interdependence of all aspects of life; the interrelationship of animal, vegetable, human food source, and chain of life-death, mirroring the universal law of impermanence and the oneness of All.

"Feeding" another person and helping another meet his or her basic need for nurturance, for food and fluid, requires a *Caritas Consciousness* of how to be in-relation, in-right-relation with self and other, present, in-the-moment, conscious, alert, aware of how to be with another. It requires an understanding, a reflective wisdom, *Caritas Consciousness,* if you will, about how to "give something to another in such a way that that person is able to receive it."

The result is the experience of nurturing, which is nourishing and reciprocal for both persons. It is through giving that we receive. The food and fluid need is associated with trust, love, warmth, and security in human relationships. Conscious and unconscious past experiences, symbolic and real meanings are associated with this basic need.

When working with another, it is necessary to have an appreciation of what eating and food mean to the person. The cultural significance of habits, familiarity of certain tastes, smells, and so on, are laden with emotions that are embodied, pre-conscious, and often unconscious.

When we are conscious of how to give to another, to minister in a loving, caring, kind way—whether formally feeding a patient unable to eat by him- or herself, giving a glass of water, or assisting one with the best dietary practices and meals—it becomes a mutual process.

This mutuality of the caring relationship in assisting another expands in a spiral toward a consciousness of all acts in which we minister/attend to another. This basic need and basic professional responsibility of assisting another with a basic human need is foundational to human caring. Helping another by attending to, helping to care for another when in need, is a sacred act of sustaining humanity and humane acts of caring.

This basic need is associated with nourishing body, mind, emotions, and spirit with food both symbolically and literally, whereby with this need we are drinking in love, friendship, companionship, support, trust, warmth, security, and so on, even in the midst of the pain, suffering, sickness, and isolation so commonly associated with illness.

SIGNIFICANCE OF THE FOOD AND
FLUID NEED FOR *CARITAS NURSING*

- Theory and research support the proposition that emotional and energetic associations are related to this biophysical basic need. Emotional factors can create associations that permeate life patterns and affect imbalances and eating disorders.

- Food and fluid need represents and symbolizes much more than the intake of nourishment for survival.

- This need is energetically associated with trust, love, warmth, security, and safety in human relationships.

- This need is related to past experiences, conscious and unconscious experiences and meanings, symbolic and real meanings associated with early feeding experiences, and relationships with food, eating, and emotional experiences with significant others.

- The cultural significance of food habits, eating practices, selection of foods, and so on, must be incorporated into a plan of caring. Familiar foods give people a sense of trust, comfort, and security.

- Food is a focus of emotional associations and interpersonal relationships. Eating habits begin in childhood from birth onward; one's culture and past experiences define for one what is edible, how and under what circumstances foods are to be eaten, savored, or valued.

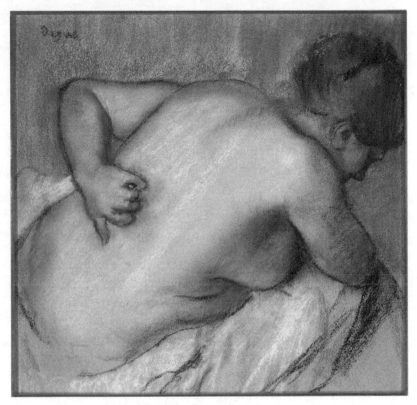

Figure 14. Femme Se Grattant, *by Edgar Hilaire Degas. Collection, The Denver Art Museum.*

- Increasingly, evolved views of food acknowledge that food is sacred and gives life force energy for human survival, honoring the sacred source of all food and water.

- The *Caritas Nurse* honors the sacred dimensions of eating and its range of symbolic and actual meanings from within the subjective experiences of the one-being-cared-for.

- In addition to Carative Factor (CF) 9 related to assisting with human needs, other CF/*Caritas Processes* with this specific need include numbers 4: developing a helping-trusting-caring relationship; 5: promoting and accepting the expression of positive and negative feelings; and 7: teaching and learning that address individual needs, styles, and readiness.

HUMAN NEED FOR ELIMINATION:
"TOILETING"/BATHING/PERSONAL APPEARANCE

If there is one major metaphor associated with being a nurse, it is the association of bedpan. The word "nursing" is often reduced to the lay association of "emptying bedpans," which is seen as a degrading act or a low level of service to another—perhaps the lowest level of work, second only to being a servant to another.

The basic need for elimination and for assistance with this need is one of the most basic bodily biological functions, but it is often laden with embarrassment, invasion of privacy, exposing of body parts, violation of one's integrity, and so on. Often, even to ask for or require help with this need is a source of anxiety, stress, inconvenience, and vulnerability for a patient.

This need not only includes the external environment required for meeting this basic bodily function but also encompasses subjective feeling states such as privacy, body image, self-image, toilet habits, patterns, and so on. However, this is a basic biological need related to health and survival. It is a necessary part of human existence.

The personal meanings associated with this broad need affect the way patients will ask for and expect assistance, when required. For example, they may delay asking for assistance; they may resist and even resent being dependent on another for help with this most basic biological function of the body. The subjective associations with this maturational need include issues of blame, guilt, money, power, and control, as well as creativity and ethical honor in relationships (Myss 1996:97).

Different cultures respond differently to basic bodily needs and functions. In the United States, social reticence is associated with this need; privacy and embarrassment are often present. Other cultures are often more open and receptive to the normal functions of the body and are not shy about needs for defecating, urinating, and sexual gratification.

A parent or an entire culture may establish values and norms related to gratification of the elimination need. As a nurse, it is helpful to understand the emotional meaning and habits of the patient in order to assist him or her. Indeed, the inner subjective feelings and meanings associated with this need may affect the normal function related to ingestion and elimination. Issues of autonomy, curiosity, shame, modesty, doubt, rigidity, and stifling or facilitating creativity all are considered to be associated with the early childhood origins and background experiences related to this need. These early feelings of giving and receiving, conforming or rebelling, are discussed in the psychodynamic literature with respect to this need.

The *Caritas Nurse* is respectful and honoring of the whole person and all the subjective meanings and associations of this need. The *Caritas Nurse* does his or her best to respond to the sensitivity of the individual.

Assisting others in meeting their basic need for cleanliness and bodily function, making themselves attractive and presentable for self and other, is critical to one's sense of self and one's sense of dignity, self-esteem, and self-regard—indeed, such basics can affect one's health and healing. Thus, this need requires skill, sensitivity, and a trusting-intimate relationship between the patient and nurse.

This need goes beyond bodily function to encompass such basic self-care needs as shaving, having a haircut, using lotions, applying makeup, and so on, that are part of a person's daily, private, personal routine. This basic routine is interrupted when one is ill and unable to carry out these tasks; thus, it is often a source of frustration, if not embarrassment and even anger, that one is dependent on another for assistance.

The sensitivity and feelings the nurse associates with this need likewise affect the nurse's response in taking care of another. Whether the need is for a bedpan or for assisting one with the daily toilet, the nurse enters into the need with a *Caritas Consciousness* that holds the other and his or her need with the utmost dignity and respect. Moreover, a reflective *Caritas Nurse* is also honoring of his or her own feelings and aware of how those feelings may interfere with care.

In caring for another with this presenting need, the *Caritas Nurse* approaches this act as a gift to the other. In fully accepting the other, in preserving the other's integrity and sensitive feelings, there is a recognition that the one receiving this assistance is deeply grateful for the dignity and honor the nurse offers through this gift of compassionate, caring service.

SIGNIFICANCE OF THE ELIMINATION NEED FOR *CARITAS NURSING*

- Subjective "feeling states" and perceptions are associated with bodily functions and physical problems with the elimination system; these perceptions and meanings are incorporated into a child's mind during early childhood development.

- Assistance with this basic human need is more than just a bio-physical function; it encompasses Martinsen's (2006) and others' existential phenomena and notions of "dwelling" as more than satisfaction of needs but rather as related to life-enhancing responses in space and place whereby one helps another find calm, rest, and dignity. This view of basic needs assistance embraces the lived experience of other and includes:
    1. Feelings of anxiety, anger, guilt, possession, resentment, control, and dependency.
    2. Societal-cultural and parental views affect early attitudes toward cleanliness, modesty, privacy, morality, immorality, and toilet habits.
    3. Experiences and meanings associated with this need during early childhood can affect self-concept, body image, and bodily functions.

- The practice of caring includes an understanding of individual desires, habits, ideas, and cultural and personal significance associated with this need.

- The foundation for this developmental stage helps promote autonomy, flexibility, curiosity, creativity; it can also affect feelings of shame, doubt, rigidity, stifling of curiosity, and inhibition of creativity.

- Assistance with this basic need is an important part of routine care for all patients. But understanding this need from a broader horizon of meaning and energetic connections with the whole person and life experiences and meanings needs to be considered in caring practices.

- In any plan of care, the *Caritas Nurse* seeks to preserve the dignity of the person and approach caring practices with the utmost respect and regard for those needing such help when they are so vulnerable and dependent upon the nurse.

- In addition to Carative Factor 9: assisting with human needs, other CF/*Caritas Processes* related to this specific need include CF/CP numbers 4: helping-trusting-caring relationship; 5: promotion and acceptance of the expression of positive and negative feelings; and 8: create a healing environment for preserving human dignity.

HUMAN NEED FOR VENTILATION: "BREATHING"

This need is full of symbolic meanings associated with breath and breathing, as well as the flow of energy throughout the body. Breathing is basic to survival, but more than just survival; our breath is the very source of life, of spirit. Through our breathing out and breathing in, breathing in and breathing out, the breath of life, we are connecting with the rhythm of the universe and the universal law of impermanence—that is, everything in the world is expanding and contracting, rising up and falling away, just like the inhalation, exhalation of the breath. We breathe in air, spirit, the breath of life. This need is associated with the heart, in that the heart, circulatory system, lungs, and diaphragm are included in the respiratory-cardiac energetic system.

The heart-lung system is associated with numerous pathological diseases—heart attacks, allergies, stress—as well as emotional conditions such as grief, anxiety, sighing, hyperventilation, and conditions such as asthma, bronchial disturbances, and other respiratory conditions. Caroline Myss (1996:99) identified "congestive heart failure, mitral valve prolapse, cardiomegaly, lung cancer, bronchial pneumonia, upper back, and shoulder and breast cancer" as physical dysfunction manifestations of the energetic anatomy of the heart area.

This basic human need includes the need for healthy air, a fresh ventilation system in one's surroundings, freedom from noxious substances and pollution, basic oxygen, and purity of the environment to ensure that the respiratory and circulatory systems are functioning. But caring for someone with this presenting need also includes preventive and ongoing practices such as relaxation, breath-work exercises, emotional release (ventilation of feelings/emotions), breathing in, and releasing.

As a natural reaction to certain circumstances, we tend to forget to breathe; we forget to exhale, holding our breath almost unconsciously.

Common expressions associated with this need remind us of its complexity and all-encompassing nature. For example, someone is said to be "holding her breath" waiting for something to happen. A variety of observations are related to different feelings and how they affect our breathing. For example, it is well-known that anxiety, anger, and resentment often result in an increased rate or decreased depth of respiration and sighing. When one is sad or dejected, a decreased rate or depth of breathing sometimes occurs. Irregular breathing is associated with anger, fear, guilt, and sadness. It is well-known that for someone who is grieving the lungs are often affected, in that there is sighing and tenseness in breathing, as if it is difficult to control one's emotions.

Anger and pent-up, repressed feelings of frustration and resentment need to be expressed constructively; if they are not, the result can be destructive release, including violent acts. Thus, nurses need to grasp the complex dimensions of this need and the strong association between emotional venting and biophysical ventilation for the heart-lung system of the body.

SIGNIFICANCE OF THE VENTILATION NEED FOR *CARITAS NURSING*

- The ventilation need encompasses respiratory and circulatory systems, the need to ventilate feelings, and sociocultural norms for releasing emotions; it is associated with the energetic anatomy of the heart area as well as the lungs and respiratory system.

- The practice of caring necessitates viewing this need within a context that includes the person's perceptions, patterns of coping, sociocultural norms, lifestyle, as well as energetic patterns and genetic and physiological demands on his or her biophysical system.

- The ability to handle emotions and feelings is a key element in maintaining health and well-being; just as oxygen, clean air, and a healthy respiratory-circulatory system are necessary for survival, so is the need to express and ventilate thoughts and feelings.

- In addition to the original Carative Factor 9 related to assisting with human needs, this specific need is highly associated with

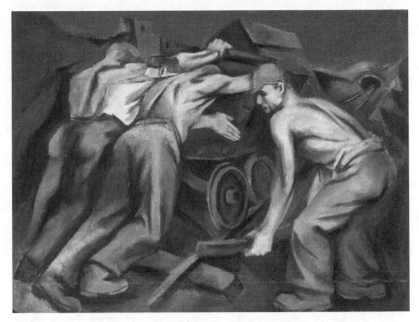

Figure 15. Mine Workers, *by Bendor Mark. Collection, The Denver Art Museum.*

CF/CP 5: promotion and acceptance of the expression of positive and negative feelings. Further, *Caritas Process* 1: practice of loving-kindness and equanimity is a foundational practice for the nurse's own health, which can be transferred directly to a caring-healing modality of breath work, relaxation, and so on, to improve healthy ventilation for patients.

- In cultivating healthy breath-work practices for self, we thus assist others in understanding the depth of this basic need and its influence on the whole person.

HUMAN NEED FOR ACTIVITY-INACTIVITY

The major questions for us . . . are: Are we doing work that serves others or generates a meaningful legacy? If not, why not? What do we want to contribute to this world? As we rediscover our interests and passions in work and service . . . we are guided, in the words of the Persian poet Rumi to "Let the beauty of what we love be [the beauty] of what we do."

ANGELES ARRIEN (2005:111)

159

A person's need for activity-inactivity is fundamental and central to one's life, as it affects the ability to move about and interact with his or her environment and to control one's external and internal surroundings. Activity and meaningful work and service through activity bring satisfaction and purposive meaning to life. Just as all human needs are holographic and each one affects the others, one's activity-inactivity need affects the ability to express oneself freely. Motion and activity are channels for expressing a broad range of emotions and abilities in the world, affecting one's behavior, lifestyle, communication, work, service, and so on.

This activity-inactivity need is connected energetically and meta-phorically/metaphysically with being "grounded" in the earth plane, in that it encompasses physical body and support. It includes the spine, legs, and feet, which are connected with one's ability to provide for life's necessities: ability to "stand up" for self. In addition, this need is physically associated with the muscular and skeletal systems.

In alignment, this need for activity-inactivity contributes physically and energetically to one's ability to trust life, to see larger patterns related to values, ethics, courage, and selflessness beyond self (Myss 1996).

The integration of this basic need is tied to personal development, learning to make choices and to take responsibility for one's actions in the world that go beyond group-mind. In other words, it is linked to the maturity to metaphorically and metaphysically "stand in place" in one's world, with coherent actions, beliefs, courage, strength, and integrity.

Activity-inactivity at the biological level channels energy constructively for efficacy, maturation, novelty, mastery, competence, and variety. In activity-inactivity, the need for relaxation, sleep, rest, reading, meditation, and so on, replenishes one's source and store of energy. Both activity and inactivity are crucial to human existence, and the expenditure of energy in ways that are nourishing, fulfilling, meaningful, and so on, is an important consideration. One wants to be cognizant of how one uses life energy; it can be channeled in ways that are restorative and replenishing, nourishing to self. Without being attentive, however, one can dribble life energy away on activities that are not meaningful or constructive for well-being.

Both action and nonaction are important for balancing one's energy with the environment. Just as breathing in–breathing out, expanding-contracting, are balancing with one's breath work, the right-relation of work-play, action-nonaction is also necessary.

The nurse is often in a caring situation in which changes in the person's activity-inactivity levels can be observed, altered, and improved. Most interventions in this area are within the nurse's realm of autonomous professional practices and clinical judgments. Changes in this need are built into the patient's plan of care, as they affect the person's healing, balance, coping, and energy balance. Whenever anyone is ill, weak, or hospitalized, there are changes in this need. Even if the person's previous tolerance for activity may have been high, engaging in the same activity in the hospital may require *more* energy.

Sometimes the patient and the nurse have different perceptions about the extent of change in activity that is necessary to promote self regulation, health, and healing. Sometimes adults and children go to extremes to demonstrate to themselves and others that they are normal and that this need is not affected by a given diagnosis or condition. For example, a friend who had chronic coronary heart disease insisted on playing vigorous games of tennis and continued to ski almost daily, even though he was aware of his diagnosis and the threat it imposed to his usual sporting activities. Indeed, he wanted consciously to live life to the fullest, even with the threat of heart attack and death, which is what he did as long as he could. He did eventually die of a heart attack, but it was as if he chose his mode of death and his style of living beyond advice from health professionals. Thus, this need, along with others, is tied up with the free will and behavior of individual patients as their meaning of living and dying. How to live a good life without restricting oneself is a philosophical, spiritual, and reality decision for each person, even at the risk of sudden death.

Any change in one's activity level necessitates a change in perception of the body's tolerance for activity-inactivity. Decisions are ultimately freewill choices on behalf of each individual. Health professionals can advise, educate, coach, and even physically assist with this basic need, especially when the person is dependent and undergoing hospitalization, incapacitation, and so on, but the level of activity-inactivity cannot be imposed or mandated for another. However, the nurse can work with the person within the context of a caring relationship and a creative problem-solving approach to help another make informed decisions for self-control, self-knowledge, self-caring, and healing acts and options. The *Caritas Nurse* seeks to identify and develop with the person the resources, ideas, objects, and acts most helpful in meeting this need.

Just as self-control over one's life and actions is critical to one's self and purpose in living, when a person's activity level is altered, the individual's self-worth is affected. The changes are often subtle and may be overlooked, as they are both objective and subjective in nature. These effects can be existential-spiritual as well as experientially real, affecting one's very being in the world. The subtle and existential changes of the sickbed experience are captured in J. H. van den Berg's "Psychology of the Sickbed."

> After a restless and disturbed sleep, I wake up in the morning, not feeling too well. I get out of bed, however, intending to start the day in the usual manner. But soon I notice that I cannot. I have a headache; I feel sick. I notice an uncontrollable urge to vomit and I deem myself so incapable of facing the day that I convince myself that I am ill. I return to the bed I just left with every intention of staying there for a while. The thermometer shows that my decision was not unreasonable. My wife's cautious inquiry whether I would like something for breakfast makes the reason much clearer. I am *really* ill. I give up my coffee and toast, as I give up everything the day was to bring, all the plans and the duties. And to prove that I am abandoning these completely I turn to the wall, nestle myself in my bed, which guarantees a comparative well-being by its warm invitation to passivity, and close my eyes. But I find that I cannot sleep.
>
> Then, slowly but surely, a change, characteristic of the sickbed, establishes itself. I hear the day begin. From downstairs the sounds of the household activities penetrate into the bedroom. The children are called for breakfast. Loud hasty voices are evidence of the fact that their owners have to go to school in a few minutes. A handkerchief has to be found, and a bookbag. Quick young legs run up and down the stairs. How familiar, and at the

same time, how utterly strange things are; how near and yet how far away they are. What I am hearing is the beginning of my daily existence, with this difference, though, that now I have no function in it. In a way I still belong completely to what happens downstairs; I take a share in the noises I hear, but at the same time everything passes me by, everything happens at a great distance. "Is Daddy ill?" a voice calls out; even at this early moment, it has ceased to consider that I can hear it. "Yes, Daddy is ill." A moment later the door opens and they come to say goodbye. They remain just as remote. The distance I measured in the sounds from downstairs appears even greater, if possible, now that they are at my bedside, with their fresh clean faces and lively gestures. Everything about them indicates the normal healthy day, the day of work and play, of street and school. The day outside the house, in which "outside" has acquired a new special meaning for me, a meaning emphasizing my exclusion.

I hear that the day has begun out in the street. It makes itself heard; cars pull away and blow their horns; and boys shout to one another. I have not heard the sound of the street like this for years, from such an enormous distance. The doorbell rings; it is the milkman, the postman, or an acquaintance; whoever it is I have nothing to do with him. The telephone rings; for a moment I try to be interested enough to listen, but again I soon submit to the inevitable, reassuring, but at the same time slightly discouraging, knowledge that I have to relinquish everything. I have ceased to belong; I have no part in it.

The world has shrunk to the size of my bedroom, or rather my bed. For even if I set foot on the floor it seems as if I am entering a *terra incognita*. Going to the bathroom is an unfriendly, slightly unreal excursion. With the feeling of coming home I pull the blankets over me. The horizon is narrowed to the edge of my bed and even this bed is not completely my domain. Apart from where I am lying it is cold and uncomfortable; the pillow only welcomes me where my head touches it. Every move is a small conquest. . . .

Change of the Future and the Past

The wallpaper which I only noticed vaguely, if I ever saw it at all, has to be painfully analyzed in lines, dots, smaller and larger figures. I feel an urge to examine the symmetrical pattern, and to see in it caricatures immensely enlarged. Hopeless and nightmarish interpretations urge themselves upon me, particularly when I am running a fever. And I feel I am going mad when I find a spot that cannot be made to fit into the structure which took me such pains to evolve.

After a few days I begin to hate the oil painting on the wall. For by this time I have acquired a certain freedom to change the caricatures of the wallpaper; I can replace the configuration I created by another one when I am bored with it. But the figures in the painting, the people, the animals, the houses and the trees, resist every attempt in this direction. The hunter, about to shoot the flying duck, remains aiming motionlessly, while I have judged his chances a hundred times. And the duck, which would probably manage to reach a hiding place if it is quick enough, defies all dangers as it comfortably floats over the landscape where the sun forgets the laws of cosmography in an eternal sunset. "Oh! Please, hurry up" I say, exasperated, and even if I am amused at my own words, I do ask the next visitor to please be kind enough either to turn the picture to the wall or to remove it altogether.

The Call of Things

As I notice my clothes, hanging over the chair at the foot of my bed, I realize with a new clarity that the horizon of my existence is narrowed. For the jacket there, the shirt and tie, belong to the outside world. I see myself descending the stairs, going to work, and receiving guests. Certainly I am that man, but at the same time, I have ceased to be him. The clothes are completely familiar and very near, and yet they belong just as truly to a world which is no longer mine. I feel a vague sympathy for these clothes, which remind me, tactfully, of my healthy existence, which must have had its value. Nevertheless, I am pleased when caring hands change my bedroom into a proper sickroom and my clothes are put away in the wardrobe. For however tactful the reminder is, I do not like to be reminded at all. After all, I cannot and will not put it into effect anyway.

If I am sensitive this way, if I possess the remarkable sense which enables people to understand the language of the lifeless objects, the discovery of my shoes is particularly revealing, even if I find it hard to put into words what these shoes, with their silent and yet expressive faces, have to say. In his famous journal [Journal II, 1935–1939 (Paris: Plon, 1939), 232], Julian Green drew our attention to the fact that it is the hat and shoes that are the most personal of our clothes. None of our clothes is entirely anonymous; they are all part of ourselves in a way, an extra skin, the skin that we choose to show others and which we want to see ourselves. We choose our various articles of clothing with this showing and seeing in mind.

A man has not very much choice in this respect. A suit is a suit; the colors may vary a bit, the material and the cut may depend on the amount of money he can afford or is willing to spend. But that is all the variety at his disposal. A man who respects himself buys a shirt that hardly differs from the one his neighbor or colleague wears. In the matter of ties we are less restricted. The salesman shows us a rainbow of colors and an array of designs. A tie can be a very personal thing. That is why we are not really pleased to find another man wearing the same tie; it seems as if we meet an attribute of ourselves which he has unlawfully appropriated.

And then the hat. Even for men the varieties in color, shape, consistency, hairiness, and handiness are almost inexhaustible. It becomes even more personal when the first newness has worn off. The hat acquires dents and creases; the brim gets a twist and a wave. These things are all signatures of the wearer and show his hold on things, his way of life. There are crying hats, proud hats, provocative hats, gloomy hats, tortured hats. And just as they tell us something about their respective owners, they certainly have something to say to their wearers themselves. Will the owner of the gloomy hat not be touched with a certain pity when he sees his hat hanging among happier members of its kind?

Shoes, too, form a very personal part of our clothing. Besides that, they enjoy the extraordinary privilege of having faces. Some shoes shake with laughter, others stare silently upon a vague distance; others again look at us full of reproach. In a store we cannot see these things yet; in their distinctive neutrality they make our choice difficult. But we have only to wear our new acquisitions a few weeks and the personality is there. As a result their faces are not unlike those of their wardrobe-mates. After all, they are of one family. Our shoes constitute our contact with the earth; they tread on country lanes and city streets. Their route is our life's course. Now they are waiting for us, there, by the bed, a silent but futile invitation. The faces with which they look at me completely explain my condition; I no longer belong to the life which nonetheless is still mine; my street, my road, lies outside the horizon of my existence.

(REPRINTED FROM J. H. VAN DEN BERG, *PSYCHOLOGY OF THE SICKBED* [1966]:23–35. BY PERMISSION OF DUQUESNE UNIVERSITY PRESS.)

Van den Berg's existential experience helps us grasp the subjective experience of a person undergoing a change in activity level as a result of sudden illness. A change in activity interferes with the person's ability to meet basic needs, to engage in daily living experiences and activities that are taken for granted. Such existential understanding of the transformation that occurs when one's activity is restricted and the person is confined elicits a very reflective, if not contemplative, view of the world, in which everything is heightened and more acute. Nightingale wrote about the importance of the nurse being aware of and attentive to small noxious stimuli such as noise, smells, and so forth, those forces that press in on someone. When one's experiential-subjective senses are confined to the sickroom and aroused by the intensity of everything slowing down, everything comes into sharper focus, to the extent that the smallest things begin to take on more significance.

Such changes lead to the need for help from another, a subjective and realistic vulnerability of having to be dependent on someone else to meet the most basic functioning required for moving through the day. When these changes occur, the person is likely to become occupied with meeting his or her needs and possibly imposing on others in an embarrassing way. Thus, the activity-inactivity need is existential, complex, and often confusing when altered.

In reality, a person is embedded in a relationship with his or her environment, with nature—with "the beauty of the forest, with the sea, the light, the sky" (Martinsen 2006:136), the mountains. With respect to the activity-inactivity need, one is connected not only with nature but also to place, including architectural space and furnishings that surround the individual, especially when considering the sickbed.

Martinsen's (2006) philosophy of life acknowledged the totality that surrounds and imbues one. It is presented as follows (from Martinsen 2006:136, referencing Bjerg 2002:50):

> One lies sick in one's Bed and feels excluded from everything, closed in, imprisoned in this constricted Room. Then one asks someone present to pull the Curtain a little to the Side. And outside are the blue, infinite Depths of the Sky, whose Waves of light have no Shore, but wash in everywhere where the Room is open, into the Heart, if it is open, and take back into those Depths all closed in Longing, unifying all the sick Singular with the eternal Whole.

As Martinsen points out, when this happens the sickroom is opened to the infinite depths of the sky, and when the heart is open, longing is set free from its imprisonment. Thus, then there is something to long for, and in this longing there is hope—the longing for life fulfillment, the feeling of being alive, different from being immobile, tied down. As this awareness filters into our view and understanding of inactivity-activity, we can honor that the human is embedded in nature, place, architecture, the room (Martinsen 2006:137), and the broader universe of the whole. When the sick, inactive, immobile person is closed in and imprisoned in the sickbed, longing and hope often do not enter; thus, one becomes more ill.

When the sickroom and the human in the room, who is ill and immobile, are turned outward to nature, the sky, a new unity of relationship with nature, place, architecture, the room, and even the larger universe is opened to the patient. "The human is unified with the whole and healing will be in this union" (Martinsen 2006:137).

Just as balanced activity is essential for living, so is inactivity. Our bodies have a biorhythmic pattern that is self-sustaining, life-energy sustaining. Our activity-inactivity level affects our efficacy and Being in the world and thus is integral with all other needs and experiences.

Even though activity and inactivity exist on a continuum of energy utilization, they have a biorhythmic pattern that is self-sustaining. There are exogenous rhythms, which depend on the external environment (e.g., seasonal variation, lunar cycles, night-and-day cycles).

Exogenous rhythms help achieve an internal balance with external stimuli. There are also endogenous rhythms, which are internal regulations. These rhythms generally function in harmony, but changes in one cycle affect the other and do not necessarily synchronize. Alternation of the waking and sleeping states is the most overt pattern of biorhythms that affects both activity and inactivity levels. A great deal of controversy and conflict exist over nurses working twelve-hour periods and switching between night and day hours for work. The biorhythms that affect levels of alertness, fatigue, social patterns, thought process, irritability, and so on, are manifest in an upsetting of one's energetic field. Activity occurs during a person's usual waking period. The waking state provides the greatest opportunity for decision making and physical activity. The sleep state provides the necessary rest and restoration required to stay in harmony with one's inner and outer rhythms of energy balance.

Just as activity is critical for one's Being-in-the-world, so is inactivity: sleep and rest. Inactivity helps one conserve and replenish energy. It helps balance the expenditure and renewal of one's source of energy. Even sleep, which is essential for energy conservation and renewal, is not passive, however. It is paradoxical that during sleep the muscles are profoundly relaxed while brain activity is increased, generally with an increase in vital signs.

This increase in cortical activity and vital signs is associated with dream states, even though the exact function of dreaming is still unknown. There are various theories to explain dreams, but some of the research validates the fact that dreams have a mental restorative function; some research indicates that it is connecting one to higher self, the unconscious, inner wisdom, one's spirit guide, and so on.

The important point here is that dreaming and sleep are critical to one's well-being. Hospitalization and sick regimes that induce interruptions of sleep lead to sleep deprivation, altered rhythms of rest-activity, and nonconstructive use of sleep, upsetting one's biorhythms.

The use of sleeping pills to address sleep deprivation often alters dream sleep and affects one's sleep pattern, accompanied by nightmares and vivid dreams that are tiring, resulting in fatigue upon awakening rather than restoration. The use of medication to help one sleep affects the quality of sleep, especially in relation to psychological and cognitive functioning. Ongoing research is occurring and needed in this area to assist nursing, scientific, and psychological knowledge relevant to this basic need.

Work is love made visible.

KAHLIL GIBRAN

SIGNIFICANCE OF THE ACTIVITY-INACTIVITY NEED FOR *CARITAS NURSING*

- The activity-inactivity need is a human need that affects all persons and experiences and events with which the nurse is involved.

- This need provides maturation, mastery, competence, variety, relaxation, and restoration.

- Inhibition of this need can thwart other human needs and cause lower-order needs to dominate.

- The more basic needs require attention to avoid usurping energy, allowing fuller actualization of other higher-consciousness needs related to creative expression, affiliation, self-actualization, and so on.

- Health changes and treatments related to illness, trauma, and life crises frequently necessitate a change in one's activity level. Any change in activity is a subjective as well as an outer experience; it can best be understood from the subjective inner-life worldview of the experiencing person, not just by external observations alone.

- The psychology involved in positively affecting the inactive sickbed is opening the room to infinite depths of nature, place, architecture, furnishings, and the room itself, related to the larger universe that helps open the human heart to be set free from imprisonment; to open one's heartfelt longing for hope, for feeling alive versus tied down, for turning outward rather than inward (Martinsen 2006).

- The practice of caring includes helping another constructively channel and balance energy among rest, sleep, and activity.

169

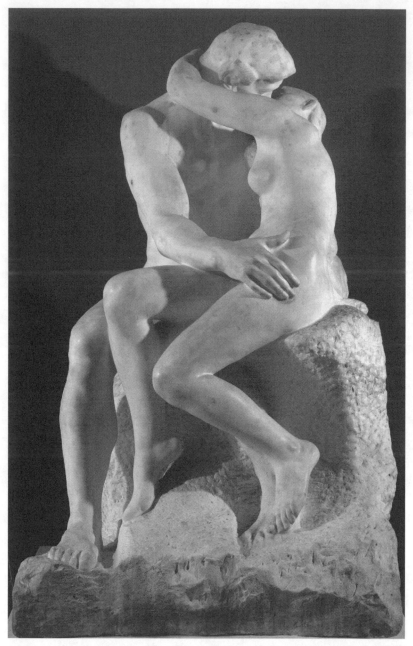

Figure 16. The Kiss, *by Auguste Rodin. Marble, 1886. Musée Rodin, Paris, France.*
Photo credit, Erich Lessing/Art Resource, New York.

- Sleep research is important for nursing and caring, in that altera-
tion in sleep patterns affects one's being-in-the-world and one's
ability to have biorhythmic balance, as well as the necessary restoration that comes from deep sleep.

- The Caring Science focus of nursing requires continual research
and development in this area; it requires utilization of available
knowledge related to this need while still fashioning the knowledge to meet the needs of the individual person.

- Finally, in addition to attending to the original Carative Factor
9: assisting with human needs, this specific need is highly associated with Carative Factor/ *Caritas Process* 6: use of a creative
problem-solving caring process, and *Caritas Process* 8: creating a
healing environment for the physical and spiritual; preserving
human dignity.

HUMAN NEED FOR SEXUALITY/CREATIVITY/INTIMACY/LOVING

Holy flesh . . .
Sacrament of intimacy; honor the love, and passion that
Brought us all
Into the world

ANONYMOUS (IN ANGELES ARRIEN 2005:71)

This need is loaded with symbolic, emotional, spiritual, and cultural
sensitivity, yet it is one of the most beautifully expressed needs, in
that our sexuality defines our identity and is an expression of our very
being. Our sexuality represents raw energy and power; it reflects the
need for an intimate union with another person with whom we can
produce and sustain life. This need invites us to "align our sexuality
and sensuality with a deep commitment to vulnerability, intimacy, and
emotional integrity, so that we may fully express the love that is in our
hearts" (Arrien 2005:75).

In an archetypal energetic model, the sexuality need is considered
to be associated with the lower-energy pelvic region of our ancient
energy system. Within the ancient energy system model of the
body, this source of sexual energy is connected to the physical body
through sexual organs, the large intestine, lower vertebrae, pelvis,
hip area, appendix, and bladder. This level of archetypical energy is

171

what grounds us in the body physical and includes not only the base instincts and needs for food and fluid and elimination but also human sexuality.

Human sexuality includes the birthing of new ideas, creativity, and self-expression at many levels. This need is energetically related not only to our human, individual inner and outer forms of expressivity of self but also to our relationship with self and our ways of relating to others. Further, this need is associated with our need to control the dynamics of our physical environment (Myss 1996). It is also associated with power, authority, and money, as well as physical, environmental, and biological forces.

Such archetypal energy enables us to generate a sense of personal identity and protective boundaries with our external world. It is the energy of self-sufficiency, our survival for being-in-the-world without having to "sell" ourselves (Myss 1996:130).

Having a mate or a life partner includes forming a union with a person of the same sex as well as having a heterogeneous relationship. The sexual expression need embodies creativity, the urge to contribute to the continuum of life. There is the expressed need to sow seeds of life, to generate matter out of energy, out of potentiality. Symbolically, this need represents our need to form sacred unions with other human beings, from which the continuation of life comes (Myss 1996).

The need for sexual expression is present in all aspects of one's being, beyond the physical, sexual act of intercourse itself. However, cheap messages from the media and marketing promote "sex" as a commodity to be bought and sold, displayed and performed, separate from any emotional-intimate loving context. This association of "sex" with object is demeaning and ultimately unfulfilling to self and other.

We violate our spirits when we fail to honor our relationship and vows to others after we have established a sacred union (Myss 1996). However, this is not to say that situations, choices, and circumstances may require that we reconsider our covenants; discord, infidelity, divorce, and separation can and do occur. As Myss (1996:82) put it: "The act of divorce [and other dissolutions] is not in itself dishonorable, but we are meant to be conscious about the manner in which we conduct ourselves during the process" of making a vow to another, whether in marriage or otherwise.

This understanding of the dynamics of this need does not mean sexual experiences, exploration, and experimentation do not and will not occur separate from a meaningful relationship. It is part of learning about oneself and accepting the feelings one has at a very basic biological level. The challenge throughout life is to honor and celebrate one's sexuality and erotic feelings within the context of a safe, loving, honoring, and intimate relationship.

Perhaps the biggest challenge with respect to our sexuality and sexual needs is learning how to honor self and all of one's being while learning to accept vulnerability, allowing oneself to be vulnerable with a trusted other, and cultivating a loving, respectful relationship and union with a meaningful other.

However, a loving, safe, intimate context and experience may be difficult to find and sustain without personal growth and self-relationship work. The ability to establish a loving, trusting, intimate sexual relationship is associated with early trusting relationships with parents. A mature sexual relationship is one that allows for risk taking in the areas of vulnerability and intimacy and Love itself.

Indeed, experiencing one's sexuality and engaging in a mature sexual relationship with another includes the ability to risk being hurt and rejected—including not being loved or wanted in a sexual relationship—without being destroyed emotionally or psychically. It also includes being able to give and receive, not engaging passively while expecting another to be responsible for your needs and fulfillment.

Learning to recognize, acknowledge, and celebrate our sexuality and sexual needs is part of the creativity of our life force and life itself. It is part of learning to live within the body we have; to accept it, love it, and appreciate it, with all its human frailties and conditions that make us human. This life force is related to self-expression, creativity, and the birthing of ideas and projects, helping connect us with honoring and accepting our own bodies and physical demands as well as our erotic and sensual needs.

Sexual expression is tied to pleasure and allows us to enjoy the full experience of human contact and release. It can be both liberating and loving. When explored and experienced without shame, the raw energy of eroticism can "elevate the human body and spirit into sensations of ecstasy, even producing altered states of consciousness at times" (Myss 1996:143). Thus, this basic human need is one to honor and celebrate, not oppress or ignore. Assisting another with honoring this basic need can be a healing act in itself, helping self and other to dwell in all aspects of one's human condition with high regard, respect, and even awe. As such, it opens up avenues for deeper levels of trust, relatedness, openness, and caring for both self and other.

SIGNIFICANCE OF THE SEXUALITY NEED FOR *CARITAS NURSING*

- The whole person is expressed through one's sexuality; sexuality is not separate from the whole person, personality, or self-expression. It is important to honor its expression as well as assess this need, along with other human needs, to help the person be-in-right-relation with self and other.

- The sexuality need is interdependent on psychological-social development as well as religious and sociocultural values, beliefs, and practices.

- Sexual gratification and fulfillment are related to a man's or a woman's confidence and pleasure in his or her self-concept and masculinity or femininity.

- Sexual fulfillment culminates and grows throughout life as one is able to enter into and sustain an intimate, loving relationship with another person.

- The essence of one's sexuality is evidenced in how one relates to self and other; sexual need and sexual expression are interwoven with one's work, play, and life force.

- Conflicting and often extreme norms and myths about sex are put forth in contemporary culture and the media. The two sexual codes considered universal are (1) the expectation and right that sexual relations will occur between marital/significant partners and (2) the prohibition against incestuous relations between parent and child and between siblings.

- Sexual behavior becomes a matter of concern for individuals or groups when it violates or is in conflict with cherished social-cultural expectations and values.

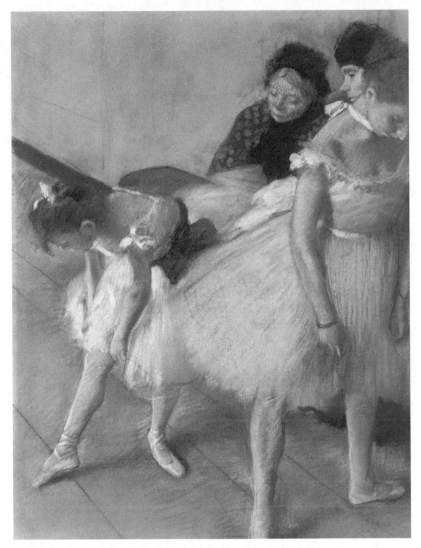

Figure 17. Examen de Danse, *by Edgar Hilaire Degas. Collection, The Denver Art Museum.*

- Society's sexual myths and stereotypes, along with the complex interaction of genes and the physiological-psychological and environmental milieu, affect the internal and external forces that comprise sexual identity, sexual expression, and so called gender differences between masculine and feminine, male and female.

175

- Sexuality expression cannot be generalized from anatomical differences between men and women; therefore, sexual need and its unique expression are perhaps best understood as a gestalt of the whole person.

- Sexuality and its expression are prominent at all stages of human growth and development. The *Caritas Nurse* is often a key person who can provide support, trust, understanding, information, guidance, and assistance with conflicting feelings, problems, and issues related to intimacy, birth control, pregnancy, parenthood, and so on, including education and stereotypes related to health-illness changes, age, and similar topics.

- The Philosophy and Science of Caring requires further study, research, and specialization in this area to contribute to the evolving knowledge regarding assistance with this basic human need.

- In addition to the Carative Factor related to assisting with basic needs generally, other Carative Factors/ *Caritas Processes* related to this specific need include number 4: developing and sustaining an authentic helping-trusting-caring relationship; 6: using creative problem solving; and 7: individualized teaching-learning.

HUMAN NEED FOR ACHIEVEMENT:
EXPRESSIVITY, WORK, CONTRIBUTING BEYOND SELF

Everyone has a longing at some level to engage in life with a sense of efficacy, work, accomplishment, and expressive achievement that contributes to the greater good, beyond self. This longing is a basic human need, and one's ability, capability, and opportunity to accomplish it contribute to self-esteem and self-actualization. This need is associated with an internal, self-defined standard of excellence that comes from within rather than without. Thus, to assess this need one has to work from the other's frame of reference with respect to standards and definitions of excellence and achievement. What may be achievement for one person may not hold for another. The outcomes of this expressivity and accomplishment are self-approval, self-acceptance, and a level of competence and achievement that satisfies oneself. Of course, indirectly, one's achievements gain approval and recognition from others; such interaction with others contributes to social graces, approval, and acknowledgment from the outer world of one's internal sense of satisfaction. However, if one's goal is outer-world achievement at the expense of what is internally meaningful, there is dissonance and a sense of meaninglessness related to our outer-world accomplishments. Without an inner motivation for self-expression, the achievement need becomes distorted or misdirected, leading to dissatisfaction, dissonance, even despair, in that there is no inner anchor for assessing the meaning if motivated solely by external forces. There is an innate motivation for behavioral competence, directionality, and purposeful striving in one's life. The need is guided by realistic expectations congruent with one's talents, gifts, and skills as well as level of maturation and readiness.

Gratification of this need is related to independent, inner-directed accomplishments and self-appraisal of those accomplishments, as well as others' appraisal of the accomplishments. It has been acknowledged in the psychological literature that biological drive alone does not explain motivation and sense of achievement. It is a subjective, psychologically complex situation related to meaning, personal interests, life experiences, self-concept, aesthetic qualities, play, exploration, and approaches to problem solving; a complex interconnection between and among cognitive-affective-behavioral experiences as well as environmental situations.

Controversy regarding gender difference continues regarding achievement and its manifestation in men and women, boys and girls. Historically, especially in Western mind-sets, women were expected to achieve in artistic pursuits, social-community interactions and roles, and more private, domestic pursuits; men were more active in business, sports, and outer-world accomplishments. In contemporary society there have been major changes in social-cultural, modern, and postmodern views of gender expectations. Thus, there is room for freedom of movement without differentiated, stereotyped mind-sets and expectations for achievements by men and women.

Views regarding achievement continue to acknowledge the complexity of interaction among competence and inner expectations; talents, skills, and values; and access to opportunities. Together these forces, combined with social norms and existing structures such as family, church, school, community groups, and organized units of society, offer a necessary reinforcement value that is internally meaningful to the individual. Rotter's (1954) early classic Social Learning Theory remains relevant. He posited:

> Behavior potential is a function of Expectation plus Reinforcement Value
> It can be framed as
> BP = f (E + RV)

Within this view, there is an understanding that a person expects that certain achievements will bring reinforcement he or she values, which in turn will satisfy an internal standard of success or accomplishment. The self-approval needed from within and without may change for a person who is ill or has an altered life situation. For example, a man who has farmed all his life may be unable to perform the degree of labor required for farming after a heart attack, surgery, and so on. Thus, his expectations of former work and achievement goals may be dramatically changed in ways that affect his self-approval, self-esteem, and inner standards.

The practice of caring often involves helping others to (1) gain a more realistic view of themselves and their expectations and (2) identify areas in which they can perform at a level they find satisfying. The opportunity structure would therefore have to be considered, as would shared social norms about expectation. Achievement is influenced by the person's expectations of success or failure in a given situation. If past achievements are no longer realistic, the person has to experience a repatterning of expectations as well as outcomes. Without a reappraisal and repatterning to create new expectations and new possibilities, a sense of low self-esteem, helplessness, hopelessness, despair, and depression can result. Compounding any personal life change in one's level of achievement are the sociocultural overlay and different values and expectations among different cultures, socioeconomic groups, geographic-climatic surroundings, and so on. Whether one is exposed to and reinforced by values and expectations of achievement or whether one is exposed to and reinforced by values and expectations of failure will contribute to achievement behaviors. Different cultures hold different values as to meanings of achievement. The Western world increasingly defines success and achievement based on money, control, and power over others and their environment, whereas other cultures and countries across time have valued and continue to value higher-order states of civilization related to artistic, literary, cultural, and spiritual accomplishments (art, music, poetry, sculpture, design, architecture, evolved human potential, a moral community, a caring society, peace, and similar values).

The achievement need is thus manifest at the individual and social-cultural levels as well as reflected among the spiritual practices of an individual, a people, a race, and a nation-state. These various dimensions, values, views, and theories of achievement need to be considered in the practice of caring.

A *Caritas Nurse* is open to explore the variety of dynamics and vicissitudes within this area as well as the potential evolution of his or her views of achievement at the individual and civilization levels. Just as self-worth and a sense of social approval are needed and desired by humans at the individual level, the same notions can hold true for nation-states and the different and meaningful forms of achievement represented by different nations, cultures, and areas of the world. Considering these matters at a higher order invites a higher level of consciousness of individual and collective action and the way these forms of action interact to affect the whole.

Within the ancient energy system, this need is related to the energetic level of the "throat" and the "third eye." It is within these energy systems that one finds issues related to choice and personal expression for using one's power to create, to follow one's dream, to pursue one's intellectual abilities, openness, ability to learn from experiences, and so on (Myss 1996).

SIGNIFICANCE OF THE ACHIEVEMENT NEED FOR *CARITAS NURSING*

- To assist with this need, *Caritas Nurses* need to understand the complex dynamics and forces operating behind the need and its different values, forms of expression at the individual and collective levels, and how it manifests at the human and civilization levels.

- It is important for *Caritas Nurses* to be cognizant of and to separate their own needs and values from what is important, expected, valued, and realistic for the one-being-cared-for.

- The *Caritas Nurse* works from the other's point of view and sub-jective human frame of reference, not exclusively from a medi-cal, professional, clinical view of expectations.

- The practice of *Caritas Nursing* includes problem solving with the other to help him or her find alternative ways to see the situ-ation, meet expectations, and seek opportunities for personal meaning, recognition, and satisfaction.

- The *Caritas Nurse* holds the person in his or her wholeness, even when previous expectations and successes need to be altered; the nurse never underestimates the person's inner motivation and potential for achievement.

- This need for achievement is affected by and affects all the other basic needs in a complex, energetic, dynamic way, so the inter-active nature of needs must be considered in an overall plan of caring.

- The other Carative Factors/*Caritas Processes* operating with this specific need include numbers 2: hope and faith; 3: nur-turing individual spiritual practices/beliefs; 4: helping-trusting caring relationship; 6: creative problem solving; and 7: teaching-learning-coaching.

HUMAN NEED FOR AFFILIATION:
BELONGING, FAMILY, SOCIAL RELATIONS, CULTURE

The Deepest need . . . is [the] need to overcome . . . separateness
And leave the prison of aloneness.

ERIC FROMM

Of all the basic human needs, the affiliation need comes closest to revealing the core of our humanity and humanness. A basic assump-tion is that people need people; this is a universal need and the basis for thriving as a human. The function of this need is *Belonging*. The matu-ration experiences are related to balancing dependence with indepen-dence, privacy with intimacy, separateness with connectedness, and individuation within the collective family of humanity.

Within the ancient energetic body system, this need can be located energetically between belonging to the whole of humanity and developing relationships, partnerships, and attachments to other people and things, learning to honor one another in our interactions. It encompasses energetic dynamics related to humanitarianism, the ability to engage in the larger pattern of life-humanity with values, ethics, and courage.

Every human being has the need to be accepted and to belong to a human group while also maintaining privacy and separateness. One's identity with group-belonging is closely related to establishing and maintaining one's own identity. One's individual distinction comes from the way a person conducts his or her own life in relation to other people. A broad consideration of this need is centered in sharing, balancing individual and group dynamics and pressures, finding self in other and vice versa, while honoring one's unique self.

An earlier theory from social psychology and sociology, referred to as the "Looking Glass Theory," posited the position: "I look in the mirror and I see myself as others see me." This is a reminder that Separation-Belonging: I-We, Me-Us constitutes a dialectical dynamic that helps define the interactive process of achieving self-identity and one's relationship with self and other. Within this context it can be explained that the affiliation need develops in response to environmental relatedness; one learns about oneself and others from the experiences from one's physical, social, behavioral, and emotional day-to-day environment and relationships.

The affiliation system allows feedback from others; this is what helps to shape one's thoughts and to support feelings, what helps one to identify and reduce anxiety. If one is deprived of this interaction, the person may fail to develop his or her potential for relatedness or become uncomfortable, withdrawn, or reclusive in interpersonal relatedness.

Gratification and maturity with affiliation provide the capacity for identification and commitment in social relatedness, allowing one to be of use in one's world. The underlying effectiveness of affiliation is tied to consistent bonding, nurturing, and attachment between mother/significant loving other and child from infancy onward.

Three interpersonal needs were identified in the early work of Schultz (1967):

1. Inclusion. The need for identity, attention, and association with others; the need to belong; the struggle about whether one is "in" or "out," alone or together, private or public. Inclusion can be associated with the original psychological notions of introversion or extroversion in different characteristics of people.

2. Control. The need for autonomy; the power to influence authority. Control also refers to decision-making processes between people. The dynamic is between controlling others or being controlled by others. It includes issues of dominance: top-bottom, dependent-independent.

3. Affection. The need for intimate, emotional relationships between and among others. These dynamics represent tension between intimacy versus isolation, whether one is close to or distant from and with other humans. Affection includes feelings of love, tenderness, acceptance, trust, warmth, and so forth; it also represents the ability to constructively handle opposite feelings, such as anger, hate, sadness, guilt, and related emotions.

These three interpersonal needs are manifest in the ancient energetic systems described by Myss (1966). She points out that the spiritual challenge of our energetic being is to learn to interact consciously with others, to form unions with people who can support our development and release relationships that handicap our growth. Within the energetic model, Myss introduces the laws of magnetism within the context of relationships: "[T]hese laws mean that we generate patterns of energy that attract people who are opposite us in some way; who have something to teach us. Nothing is random; prior to every relationship we have ever formed, we opened the door with energy that we were generating. . . . The more conscious we become, the more consciously we can utilize the energy" (Myss 1996:132).

Myss says that in every relationship there is a primary conflict of faith and choice: relationships generate conflict and conflict generates choice. We break free when we learn to transcend the dualism between others and ourselves (we are all connected at the human spirit level) and transcend the dualism between God and ourselves. Myss (1996:135) reminds us that as long as we focus on trying to control another person and forget that that person is a mirror reflecting back to us our own qualities, we keep conflict alive. Seeing self and others in "right-relation," through symbolic connections for shared learning, we learn to accommodate differences. This provides the foundation for the deeper notion of communion, going beyond superficial affiliation as a collection of interpersonal relationships.

Likewise, the energetic system involved with this need is related to creative energy and the desire to contribute to the continuum of life. This creative energy helps us break habitual patterns of relationships, helping to reshape and repattern the chaos of our world and our relationships (Myss 1996). Beyond our intimate personal relationships, there is the affiliation with relationships outside the primary family. These include extra-familial groups in the community (church, school, peers, colleagues, neighbors, and business, social, and recreational contacts).

These extra-familial relationships include (1) forming friendships with others; and (2) sharing, associating, working, and joining with others. These interactions lead to humanitarian service through community, civic, professional, religious, and charitable organizations. They allow one to extend oneself beyond one's immediate self. These characteristics are related to altruism and caring for others, previous and future generations. Without relationships, humans lose contact with reality and the social nourishment necessary for survival. The opposite of affiliation is isolation.

Reports across time and experiences highlight what happens to people if they are isolated from other humans:

1. The "pain" of isolation: prisoners of war have reported that they prefer torture to isolation from others.

2. People exhibit a strong tendency to dream, think, fantasize, and occasionally hallucinate about others.

3. They experience withdrawal, suffering, apathy, diminished growth and development, and even failure to thrive.

This basic need is affected by any health-illness situation. When a person is worried about his or her health or is actually ill, the individual often has decreased contact with others, including the family or primary support system as well as significant others. Decreased feelings of belonging can result from such withdrawal or disengagement, even though it may be a necessary coping process.

This gradual but real disengagement as a result of illness was captured in the previous section on the need for activity and the existential story of van den Berg. The excerpt is relevant to understand how the affiliation need is affected by even a minor illness and being in a "sickbed." The sickbed, or form of isolation resulting from illness, leads to loss of contact with day-to-day activities and routines, deprivation and disruption of patterned behaviors and experiences we take for granted. Suddenly, when life patterns are interrupted, there is a surreal sense involving even intimate relationships and familiar activities that previously were commonplace; they become estranged and distant, even foreign, to the sick person.

Regardless of the life situation that triggers isolation from affiliation (e.g., worry, illness, diagnosis, loss, change, fear, trauma, and so on), when a person's capacity to focus on others is reduced, his or her usual affiliation needs change, resulting in frustration. At the same time, when one's affiliation is compromised, there tends to be a need for a quantitative decrease of relationships—a desire for fewer people around the person; one's social space and social sphere contract. Correspondingly, there is a qualitative increase in the value of the people who are around the individual. Having fewer people around who are special, close, intimate, and meaningful may be more satisfying than having many people who may have only a superficial connection to the person.

A hospitalized person may be denied the few qualitative relationships he or she needs and desires and instead may have more limited superficial relationships with a variety of often impersonal visitors or, worse still, impersonal, detached caregivers: "They have swabbed me clean of my loving associations" (Sylvia Plath).

Nurses are often the ones who affect the quality of interactions with persons during illness; therefore, nurses and *Caritas Nursing* are vital in assisting with the affiliation need. Such awareness and understanding of this need at many levels are necessary to guide caring practices.

SIGNIFICANCE OF THE AFFILIATION NEED FOR *CARITAS NURSING*

- The need for affiliation is a universal human need and it forms the core of humanism.

- This need is the basis for one's cooperative undertakings with others in the world and the foundation for relating to self and others.

- Affiliation behaviors are manifested differently by different people on a continuum of privacy-separation of oneself to intimacy and closeness with others. This is a learned process through cooperative experiences, interactions, and participation.

- The primary group family best provides the relationship and environment necessary for development of this need.

- The affiliation need and its manifestation are affected by health-illness changes, hospitalization, and treatment regimes.

- During health-illness changes, a person has a reduced capacity for others and a heightened need for quality relationships over quantity of relationships.

- The Carative Factors / *Caritas Processes* that accompany this specific need most prominently are numbers 4: developing helping-trusting-caring relationships and 6: creative problem solving.

HUMAN NEED FOR SELF-ACTUALIZATION/SPIRITUAL GROWTH

Modern mainstream personality theories have acknowledged that every human being has an internal striving to become, to grow, to fulfill self. This striving is referred to commonly as the need for self-actualization. It is considered a universal human need and is manifest in unique ways.

As Siddhartha expressed it (Hesse 1951:31): "[W]hat was it they could not teach you? And he thought: It was the Self, the character and nature of which I wished to learn. . . . Truly nothing in the world has occupied my thoughts as much as the Self . . . that I am one and am separated and different from everybody else, that I am Siddhartha."

This reference reflects the reality that every person in certain respects is:

1. Like all other persons (universal)

2. Like some other persons (group)

3. Like no other person (unique). (Kluckholn, Murray, and Schneider 1953:53)

This focus points out the internal need for each person to mature to the highest level of self as an innate striving. Values inherent to self-actualization are related to inner meanings rather than to facts alone. Perhaps it is more relevant to think of this need as an individual continuum along an inner self-defined movement; each individual determines how far to seek fulfillment, with wide individual differences. These differences are related to a complex of past and present experiences as well as successes along the way with other needs and desires for self and one's being-in-the-world. Some persons are more achievement-oriented than others, which intersects with this need; however, striving for self-actualization is closer to the birthing of the inner spirit and its fuller, unique emergence.

While self-actualization is motivated internally, it is affected by one's external environment, often requiring a change externally to repattern for more harmony of mind-body-spirit, Oneness-of-Being. However, for one to "be-in-right-relation with self" may require changes in relationships with others.

The concept of self-actualization in a conventional sense applies to the mature adult. According to the work of Erikson (1963), the self-actualized person is one who elevates his or her consciousness to higher cultural, ethical, and spiritual levels. This conception includes the notion of *generativity*—that is, an ecologically supportive environment for human caring and health for future generations as well as the entire human species. Thus, a self-actualized person is concerned with problems outside of and beyond self, with a mission in life for an internally oriented task to fulfill, a task that helps establish and guide the next generation toward human and environmental health.

At the same time, it is idealistic and perhaps unrealistic for everyone to evolve toward their highest level, in that we are all here on the earth plane for our own experiences and purposes, and each person has his or her own path to follow. However, this reality still allows the

Caritas Consciousness Nurse to hold others in their highest ethical sense of Being and Becoming, even if they cannot see it for themselves at the moment. An awareness of this human need invites each of us, whether nurse or patient, to listen and open to the inner call to follow one's authentic inner self in the outer world.

This need thus intersects energetically with evolving consciousness and is consistent with Newman's notion of "health as evolving consciousness" (Newman 1994). Quality of living is associated with self-love, self-awareness, and self-knowledge—allowing for more self-caring, self-healing, self-knowledge, and self-control through insightful, informed choices, decisions, and actions. This evolving awareness provides one with the ability to face life more directly, with its pain, joys, sorrows, and suffering as well as challenges, opportunities, and successes. Our evolving consciousness contributes to our understanding of life patterns and stresses and how they contribute to our well-being or illness and disease.

SIGNIFICANCE OF THE
SELF-ACTUALIZATION NEED FOR *CARITAS NURSING*

The notion of self-actualization placed within a contemporary energetic *Caritas* framework invites other considerations that make new and broader connections between the inner and outer in self-development and between the human and the universe that go beyond the conventional separatist mind-sets of the Western world—that is, the prevailing mind-set that pits humans against each other, their environment, planet Earth, and the larger universe that is our shared home. The energetic mental field of consciousness is the entry point that "pours endlessly into the human energy system, from the greater universe, from God or the Tao" (Myss 1996:265).

By locating ourselves within the dominant view that separates self from our spiritual-evolved consciousness dimension, except in private personal matters, we find ourselves in a conflicted world of practice and human evolution. On the one hand, the world is filled with spiritual awareness, from Florence Nightingale forward; on the other hand, the public world favors exclusivity of the physical plane, leading to conflict, blame, and violence, wars against and over each other.

Thus, we all are simultaneously caught in a worldview or cosmology that continues to place sovereignty over external aspects of the material and natural worlds, disconnecting us from our shared humanity in the universe.

We need a larger cosmology to allow for both private and personal self-actualization and to connect with and open to the energy of God consciousness, evolving consciousness, referred to as the spiritual connector (Myss 1996).

Our recent history in an evolving Western culture allows for abundant private and personal self-actualization efforts. We see, for example, a multitude of spiritual practices in the areas of self-growth and self-awareness pursuits, for example:

> [E]thical service and humanitarian compassion, an inward turn toward meditation, prayer, monastic withdrawal, spiritual pilgrimages, involvement with great mystical traditions and practices from Asia (Hindu, Buddhist, Taoist, Sufi), and diverse indigenous and shamanic cultures (Native North American, Central and South American, African, Australian, Polynesian, Old Europe). Recovery of various Gnostic and esoteric perspectives and practices . . . devotion to creative, artistic expression as a spiritual path, or renewed engagement with revitalized forms of Jewish and Christian mysticism, traditions, beliefs, and practices. (Tarnas 2006:31)

At the same time, these practices and personal pursuits for deepening our humanity and the human evolutionary experience are "taking place in a cosmos whose basic parameters have been defined by the determinedly non-spiritual epistemology and ontology of modern science" (Tarnas 2006:31). In this dominant focus, these very rich, noble, human spiritual pursuits are pursued in a universe whose nature it is "to be supremely indifferent to these very quests" (Tarnas 2006:31).

This is a dilemma not only for the evolved human but also for humanity and the cosmos. It is and has been one of the unnamed dilemmas of modern nursing. As Richard Tarnas (2006:31) put it: "The very nature of the *objective* universe turns any spiritual faith and ideals into courageous acts of *subjectivity,* constantly vulnerable to intellectual negation" [original emphasis]. Put another way, both the contemporary soul and our evolving consciousness pursuits of self-actualization (which are ultimately spiritual in nature) "live within us fully yet anti-thetically. An impossible set of opposites thereby resides deep in the modern sensibility" (Tarnas 2006:30) and within each of us.

Modern life is characterized by fundamental conflicts between religious worldviews that see humans as spiritual beings in a meaningful cosmos and a scientistic worldview that sees physical matter and physical energy as the only reality.

CHARLES TART (QUOTED IN VAUGHN 1995:29)

Thus, the human need for self-actualization, spiritual evolution, spiritual fulfillment, evolving consciousness for transcendence, and higher connections is complicated by an outer world that is material and secular at its core. A new worldview or cosmos is upon us at this point in human history. We are all on a journey toward an evolving consciousness that is opening to an exploration of a vast spiritual universe of many paths that lead to wholeness, from fear to love and from material bondage to wisdom and inner freedom (Vaughn 1995).

This awakening from the Heart center, energetically moving upward in the body system, is the path of a *Caritas Nurse* and *Caritas Nursing*; this path integrates the shadow and light sides of our deep humanity, the joy and suffering side by side, not denying any part of the human experience to which we all belong. We as a civilization at this point in human history must awaken to a new cosmology and worldview that can be referred to as a Universal Heart—a universe that is a spirit-filled energy consciousness to which we all belong and have our being; a universe that is interdependent, connecting everything and us; a universe alive and evolving in harmony with each of us on the path of awakening. So, to repeat: what we hold in our hearts matters and affects our own evolution and that of humanity itself.

As developed in more depth in *Caring Science as Sacred Science* (Watson 2005), a model of Caring Science creates open heart space to connect the ethic and infinity of Cosmic Love, allowing for the inner and infinite nature of our reality to emerge and be present with respect to our Being and Belonging to the wider universe. In this work and world of Caring Science and *Caritas Nursing*, we are not restricted to the outer,

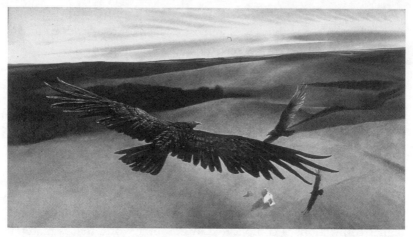

Figure 18. Soaring, *by Andrew Wyeth. Collection, Shelburne Museum, Shelburne, Vermont.*

physical world alone; that was the science model of a past era, which cut our humanity off from its life source and cut the heart and soul out of our personal and professional lives and work (Watson 2005).

> As we examine the truth of Belonging-Being-Knowing and Doing our caring-healing work in the world, how can we any longer bear to sustain and perpetuate an empty, hollow model? Especially once we honor and acknowledge our participation with the infinity and the mystery of healing and life itself? This evolving model of Caring Science opens science and our knowing to its Source—not its separation—from the knowable and unknowable to a wisdom that knows and honors/surrenders to the differences. (Watson 2005:67)

Now we reenter a new space in which there is once again room for miracles in our life and work and world. This era in Caring Science is a time for reenchantment of the wonders, the unknowns, the mysteries of the universe, awakening the heart as well as the wisdom-seeking mind, beyond knowledge itself. Such an opening in our worldview takes us to the last Carative Factor/*Caritas Process.*

CHAPTER FIFTEEN

From **CARATIVE FACTOR 10:** *Allowance for*
Existential-Phenomenological Forces
to **CARITAS PROCESS 10:** *Opening and*
Attending to Spiritual/Mysterious and Existential
*Unknowns of Life-Death**

As for me, I believe in nothing but miracles.

WALT WHITMAN

This factor in the original (1979) work is perhaps the most difficult one
for people to grasp, in part because of the language and terms. All I
am trying to say is that our rational minds and modern science do not
have all the answers to life and death and all the human conditions we
face; thus, we have to be open to unknowns we cannot control, even
allowing for what we may consider a "miracle" to enter our life and
work. This process also acknowledges that the subjective world of the
inner-life experiences of self and other is ultimately a phenomenon,
an ineffable mystery, affected by many, many factors that can never be
fully explained.

---

* Phrase "allowing for a miracle" courtesy of Resurrection Health, Chicago.

We live in a world in which we can invite new views of science, art, spirituality, and the mystery of life back into our world. A Caring Science framework acknowledges that we ultimately dwell in mystery; life is not a problem to be solved but a mystery to be lived; human problems reside in ambiguity, paradox, and impermanence; suffering, healing, miraculous cures, synchronicity are all part of the dynamic of vibrating possibilities in our evolved consciousness. Thus, within the *Caritas Consciousness* Model of Nursing, the nurse is open to what Resurrection Health called "allowing for a miracle," whereby the *Caritas Nurse* holds the patient's hope for a miracle. The *Caritas Nurse* is open to other happenings at a higher order even in the midst of modern science and concrete treatment; thus, he or she is always open to the mystery of a deeper order of the universe unfolding within a bigger picture than the human mind.

This Carative Factor/*Caritas Process* honors the reality that when anyone has a major life change, the person returns home evoking at a deep level an existential-spiritual crisis. A sudden life change as a result of a new diagnosis, illness, trauma, or abrupt life-death circumstance requires a total reexamination of one's life: questions arise as to what is most important. What are one's priorities? What matters when one has to stop midstep in the midst of one's usual life? These questions are existential-spiritual in nature and are responded to based on the experiencing person's phenomenological life view. Everyone responds differently depending on their experiences, values, belief system, perceptions, the meaning of the condition, situation, support systems, courage, determination, and so on—all of which give them the strength to face life and its vicissitudes of change and impermanence.

The personal struggles and inner crises of experiencing suffering and turmoil in one's life and health do not fit into any categories of modern medical science; they are existential and unknown in nature, unique to that individual and his or her life circumstances. It is Caring Science, not medical science, that can offer another way to view humanity and the human condition of Being-in-the-world; to look at and into the inner-life world through the other person's eyes, not through a medical science lens. For it is only through a broader, more existential-spiritual lens that we can surrender to the mysteries of human life and human predicaments. Many people have experienced tragedies in living and dying; often, these instances bring profound depth and meaning to one's life rather than the shallowness and superficiality of a diminished level of living in the material plane alone.

Such profundity of living is shown in the existential-spiritual struggles of Viktor Frankl (Frankl 1963). As a prisoner in a concentration camp for a long period of time, he struggled to find a reason to live after his release. His entire family, except for his sister, had died in the camps. He lost every possession, had every value attacked, had suffered from hunger, cold, brutality, and fear of extermination. Yet he was able to find a deeper meaning and responsibility in his life that transcended his sorrows and suffering.

In contrast to Frankl's involuntary suffering and his search for deeper meaning is the example of Leo Tolstoy. He had an aristocratic life of luxury and wealth but voluntarily subjected himself to suffering, deprivation, and isolation to find meaning and responsibility in his life. Although Tolstoy's philosophy was not considered existential at the time in that it was more a spiritual quest, the beliefs he held in the early 1800s are closely related to the later existential views of Sartre (1956), Heidegger (1962), Buber (1958), and others. Thus, we see the overlap between and among existential and spiritual questioning and quests in the human search for meaning.

These notions of existentialism, phenomenology, and spirituality are closely related and support a subjective appreciation of the inner-life world of the experiencing person, as well as an appreciation for the mysteries, multiple meanings, and unknowns of life. This *Caritas Process* invites an opening to allowance for mysteries, miracles, and a higher, deeper order of life's phenomena that cannot be understood with the ordinary mind and mind-set. In other words, the outer appearance or behavior of what is happening to another in the outer world may not necessarily reflect the inner subjective unknowns or deeper dimensions of the larger universe. Acknowledging and incorporating this *Caritas Process* into nurses' understanding of practice can be a guiding influence and a turning point for healing, whereby a tragedy can turn into a miracle of courage and strength, opening to another reality of life's deep meaning.

THE EVOLVED *CARITAS NURSE*

Once we incorporate evolving consciousness awareness into our frame of reference, including the interconnectedness of the ancient energetic body system, we open to the wider universe in awe and wonder. As nurses and the human community move energetically into heart space, we move closer and closer to our spiritual nature and to connecting with the infinite source of universal Love. As we progress and evolve toward this deeper awareness, we come closer to honoring the sacred, the higher spirit of the universe, as an integral part of our lives. We use these deeper connections to guide us.

We open our hearts and minds to seek a deeper, more intimate relationship with that which is greater than self, the Divine. We open to prayer, to humility, to asking for what we need from the larger universe through acts of faith and hope. We once again open to the transcendent dimension of living and dying, beyond the physical body localized in the material plane alone. This *Caritas Process* awakens us energetically to seek devotion, inspirational words, affirmations, prophetic beliefs, mystical and miraculous connections and ideas. It is aligned most directly with the highest energy source of cosmic Love, which honors a spiritual awakening, moving us beyond the group mind to connect consciously and intentionally with that which is greater—God, the Divine—allowing for miracles as well as mystical transcendent experiences; overcoming loneliness, isolation, even madness when faced with that which is considered unbearable. Through this *Caritas Process* and grasping its meaning we learn how to understand that the human learns how to bear the unbearable through this awakening connection. The result not only can be transformative in moving through the dark night of the soul, but also it can lead to profound insights, depths of gratitude, and appreciation of all one is learning through the journey of life itself: the joy, pain, and everything. One can also experience profound bliss, blessings, and inner peace once one is capable of surrendering to these deeper connections in the midst of darkness, fear, and despair. It is in this space that miracles can and do occur and people report experiences with angels and other happenings beyond the ordinary realm of existence.

In summary, nursing as a profession daily confronts special circumstances and people's struggles with their own Being and the meaning of the human predicaments of life and death, the challenges and realities of life-death crises of existence in between ordinary life passages. Everyone has a personal story about his or her experiences and predicaments. Each person seeks his or her own meanings to find inner peace and right-relation in the midst of fear, hatred, threats, doubts, despair, and unknowns.

These situations and experiences that face the nurse invite the nurse-self to confront her or his own state of meaning, of *Being* and *Non-Being*. When a person is able to explore her or his own existence and evolving consciousness for maturity in engaging in the vicissitudes of life and death, the individual's heart is opened to more compassion, awe, dignity, and respect for unknowns; we become more mature, more real, and more authentic to self and others in our personal and professional life. We open to previously unrecognized sources for hope, courage, power, and miraculous happenings in our life as well as in the lives of others.

Consideration of and openness to this dimension of nursing may be the most fulfilling aspect of practice. Explanatory notions of this aspect of nursing not only are best understood from an existential-spiritual-phenomenological lens but perhaps are only understood from this higher plane of seeing the world.

CONCLUSIONS

The *Caritas Nurse/Caritas Nursing*

This model of nursing is not for every nurse. It is an invitation to nurses who seek a deeper dimension of their work and calling in their caring and healing practices. In recent years there have been calls for nursing to renew itself. One aspect of such renewal comes from renewal of the spirit. The last Carative Factor/*Caritas Process* addresses this renewal of the spirit of self and system by attending to this awareness, this awakening. This revised book, *The Philosophy and Science of Caring*, goes beyond models of health-illness and disease. It aligns nursing and its authentic mission of health-healing with a deeper humanitarian and spiritual cause; that cause is about helping to sustain humanity itself, contributing to the evolution of humankind toward more spirit-filled beings connected with the infinite field

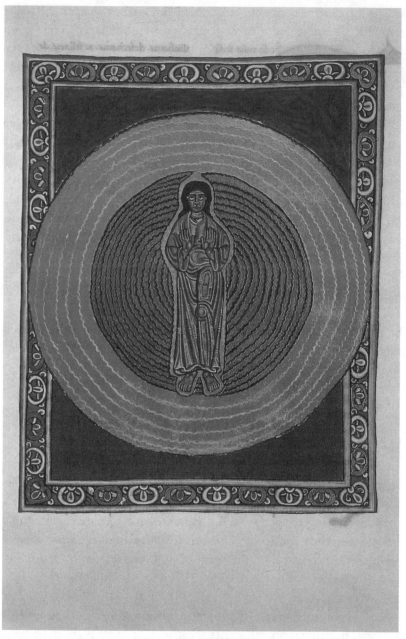

Figure 19. Holy Trinity, *by Hildegard of Bingen. From* Illuminations of Hildegard of Bingen, © *Otto Müller Verlag, Salzburg, 1954.*

of universal Love (Watson 2005). This work is ultimately about translating a deep ethic, an authentic value system, along with theory and knowledge, into living and breathing models of caring and healing in the world and in our daily work.

Thus, in positing nursing within this evolved work and world of healing, we are contributing to the healing of self and others, evolving toward a moral community; this evolution aligns human caring and healing with peace. We do not do this by some grand scheme "out there" or in a theory textbook, in some distant fantasy model. We live it in our daily practice, our moment-to-moment encounters with self and other. We do it through a disciplined approach to our personal practice, which in turn becomes a more mature professional model accessing the energetic connections of human-universe as part of our evolution.

In this *Caritas Model* of Nursing as the Philosophy and Science of Caring, we can identify at least two types of service to humanity:

1. Overt service—the outer world of clinical practice at the body-physical, material-technological level of medical services, tasks, procedures, and so on. This level of so-called ordinary or regular nursing would work from a consciousness that focuses more on the base energetic, physical body system with an unreflective ego mind-set.

2. Subtle service—the inner world of practice at the heart level, evolving toward a higher consciousness that cultivates an awakening of the heart and mind, embracing the finest of the medicalized, technical outer world while consciously cultivating the subtle inner practices of evolving our own humanity. We learn that we are *Being* and *Becoming* the *Caritas-Communitas* field, informing practices in our daily life that contribute to a collectively evolving spiritual *Caritas Consciousness*. As nurses individually and collectively engage in *Caritas Consciousness,* they become the magnetic field of attraction for others, offering a new field of compassion and a calming, soothing, loving presence in the midst of life threats and despair.

This view of "Being the *Caritas* Field" for caring and healing, which embraces both overt and subtle practices, is transformative for self and other. This is the noble work for humanity itself within an ancient and noble profession; it aligns nursing with its true mission of sustaining humanity from within and without the medical system. This new evolved form of nursing can be considered *Caritas Nursing*, Energy Nursing, Transpersonal Nursing, Holistic Nursing, Contemplative Nursing, and so on. Whatever it is named, it goes beyond ordinary nursing and sets a new and higher standard of excellence for caring, healing, and peace in the world.

Lee Kaiser, a health futurist and visionary, has said that "nurses of the future will be hired because of their caring consciousness" (Kaiser personal communication, 1989). The level of development of *Caritas Nursing* described in this book gives new meaning to his projections.

Whatever this evolved nurse/nursing is called, it offers a hopeful paradigm and vision for humanity, for health, for humans and all living things, for a living planet and universe in which we are co-creating our own destiny and future. This is the ultimate future for nurses' full contribution to society. As nursing enters this new, deep transformative field of *Caritas* practices, we each enter an entirely different new world for the new millennium unfolding before us.

This *Caritas Consciousness* evolution also requires a new language: an alchemical, transformative, nonmedical, nonclinical language. Caring/Love/*Caritas* is not sentimental but taps into our connection with the infinite field of healing Love. It is not that we dismiss the overt outer world and its empirical, clinical, technical language; it is that we realize that the two different language systems vibrate at a different level. We are at a point in our human and disciplinary maturity that we can admit and embrace new languages of beauty, poise, grace, charm, mercy, miracles, mystery, and so on. We need language and discourses that vibrate at a higher frequency, that stretch us into new depths of meaning, new evocative understandings, metaphors, myths, stories, and wise images that conventional, outer technical worlds and words cannot convey but that are needed to touch the deeply human dimensions of our world.

The word "Nurse" may be one such word with paradoxical vibrations. It operates in both the overt and subtle energetic worlds and words. It is more established and developed in the overt material model of outer basic energetic work; it has yet to cultivate the language and actions that reflect the next evolution and mature *Caritas Nursing*, which reflects the subtle energetic field of *Caritas*. Yet this subtle evolutionary practice of nursing may be the hope for nursing's authentic survival; this level of nursing is a very different quality of nursing from that commonly known in the twentieth century. The evolved *Caritas Nurse* turns to "things of spirit" as well as material form.

When nursing individually and collectively engages in caring and healing practices at this higher-deeper, subtle but powerful vibratory level, we will turn to words and actions that vibrate at a higher level— words and actions that nurture Spirit and the human soul of our work. We turn to, for example:

Beauty

Silence

Nature—other living things

Arts

Music-Sound

Relationships

Personal Story—literature-drama-film-narratives

Movement-Dance

Prayer

Meditation

Mystery—metaphors

Miracles

Infinity of Universal Love—opening to Miracles

Grace and Mercy of life and all its gifts

God

PART IV

Expanding Knowledge-Building Frameworks for Reconsidering
Caritas Nursing: *The Energetic Chakra-Quadrant Model*

CHAPTER SIXTEEN

Integral Model for Grasping Needs in Caritas Nursing

The Church says: The body is a sin.
Science says: The body is a machine.
Advertising says: The body is a business.
The body says: I am a fiesta.

EDUARDO GALEANO, *WALKING WORDS* (QUOTED IN ARRIEN 2005:77)

As discussed in previous work (Watson 2005), Wilber's Integral Model (Wilber 1998, 2001a, 2001b) provides a Caring Science / *Caritas* context for grasping the totality of a broader disciplinary focus for providing views of the body and thus basic nursing care. In Wilber's Four-Quadrant Integral Model we move toward greater depth to comprehend multiple ways of Knowing and Being and Becoming—an approach that integrates and includes subtle and dense matter, body, soul, and Spirit (Wilber 1998:102). This model seeks to point toward

Table 16.1 Wilber's Four-Quadrant Model (from Wilber 1998)

Interior: Upper left	*Exterior: Upper right*
Subjective meaning–inner-life world; phenomenological view; incorporates spirit realm "I" Knowledge / Knowing Location of intentionality, interpretive consciousness, and often unmeasurable realm of invisible inner states of mind, thoughts, consciousness	Objective-external physical world Outer-world information, measurement Judgments of observations "It" Knowledge / Knowing Location of behavioral, she / he biological observable realm
Interior / Intersubjective / Collective: Lower left	*Interobjective / Exterior Collective: Lower right*
Collective meaning; social, cultural norms "We" Knowledge / Knowing "Our" (tribal-group) perspective, interior We / Our; invisible web of worldviews, morals, religion, spiritual beliefs, myths, archetypes, magic realm Symbolic meanings, historic influences, metaphoric associations	Social-community outer-world views "It"–"They" Knowledge / Knowing Visible norms, communal, environment, social systems Collective behaviors of group, family (professions), village, nation-state, planetary

integration of the immanent with the transcendent-transpersonal, the sacred with the ordinary (Watson 2005).

The four-quadrant model offers a framework for most basic views of subjective / objective, individual / collective, insider / outsider templates for understanding core components of a given process, phenomenon, or practice at a given point in time.

Within Wilber's integral framework, he acknowledges that we need knowledge and practices in all four quadrants. However, within the practice arena, nursing has historically tended to locate itself professionally with the right side of the quadrant, while within the academic world, some of the most rapidly evolving disciplinary-theoretical work tends to lean toward the left side of the quadrant.

In reality, we need the integral, comprehensive approach for Caring Science and notions of *Caritas* practitioners. This broader framework acknowledges and systematically allows for all ways of knowing as well as for evolving ways of knowing yet to be named and explored (Jarrin 2006), allowing for different levels of development, different levels of consciousness evolution, different intelligences—moral and emotional as well as intellectual—and so on. For nursing, this development allows us to embrace knowledge and knowing in a variety of ways—those objectively known and those approaches yet to emerge from the nonphysical sphere.

For example, with an understanding of the different spheres/quadrants of knowing, we can accommodate nursing diagnosis/taxonomy and concrete physical-technical procedural acts on the one hand with the spiritual and philosophical, subjective, intentional, symbolic, Caring/*Caritas Consciousness*, "Presencing," and Being on the other hand. As Jarrin (2006) noted in an exposition of a unifying theory of nursing, such nursing has a unifying core for understanding and translating different foci of nursing within the quadrant context. Thus, nursing is more able to communicate between and among different foci and through the different and diverse lenses nursing and nurses bring to the academic and professional practice world. This shift toward integration of the whole, allowing for different conceptualizations, unites rather than separates the many diverse levels and discourses within the field.

It is within this broader and deeper aspect of tending to basic needs that we realize that nursing is simultaneously touching upon or mediating all aspects/quadrants and all energetic chakra system levels, either intentionally or unintentionally. Thus, it is important to be more intentional, aware, and evolved with respect to where we locate or "situate" (Jarrin 2006) our caring practices with respect to this *Caritas Process* of basic human needs. Chapter 17 explores the seven chakra systems as another overlay of the quadrant model, consistent with Caring Science and *Caritas Nursing*.

CHAPTER SEVENTEEN

*The Seven Chakras: An Evolving Unitary View of the Basic
Needs Energy System*

The ancient archetypal Eastern chakra system of energy anatomy or
power centers of the human energy system comes into play in deepening our understanding of basic needs and how to assist another
with his or her basic needs. This view goes beyond Maslow's (1968)
Hierarchy of Needs Model and incorporates both physical and nonphysical needs as one integrated energetic system. This ancient
yet evolved energetic chakra system can be seen as an overlay on
the Wilber Integral Quadrant Model. It invites the more advanced
Caritas Consciousness Nurse to move from focusing exclusively on
the dominant right side of the quadrant and prepare for more intentional, conscious caring-healing acts and practices that originate in
the left quadrant but manifest in the right, outer-world quadrant.
An introduction and overview of the chakra system will help clarify
this view.

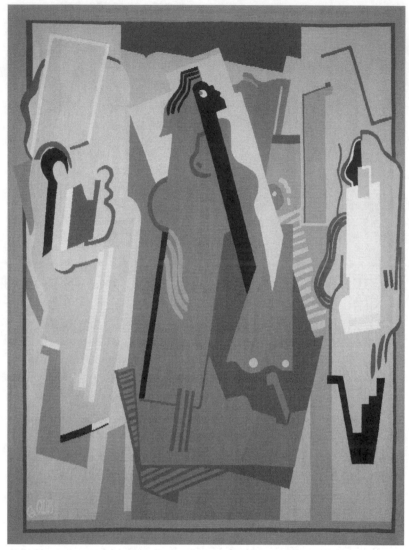

Figure 20. Autorité Spirituelle et Pourvoir-Aubusson, *by Albert Gliezes. Collection, The Denver Art Museum.*

In the chakra energetic body system, there are seven centers of power, or life force centers, that run through our bodies. However, within this system of knowledge there is a oneness of biological, psychological, emotional, and spiritual needs; they are all the same. For example, in this energetic body system model, spirituality is an inherent biological need, just as biological needs for food and fluid, elimination, and ventilation are inherently spiritual (Myss 1996).

Perhaps within this non-dual holographic integration of Wilber and Myss (Four-Quadrant Model with Seven-Center Energetic Chakra System), with respect to *Caritas Nursing* and basic needs we can envision chakras as what Wilber refers to as "lines" of development and states of caring that transcend the quadrants, running through them. Jarrin (2006) uses examples of such lines in nursing as:

- Roach's Six Cs of Caring (Roach 2002)
- Watson's Clinical *Caritas Processes* (Watson 2004a)
- Leininger's Taxonomy of Caring Constructs (Leininger 1981).

Newman's (1994) theory of health as expanding consciousness, Rogers's (1970) Unitary perspective, Boykin and Schoenhofer's (2001) ontological caring stance, and Watson's (2002a, 2003, 2005, 2006) transpersonal writings account for nonphysical, nonordinary states in caring. Thus, different types of caring can include professional (nursing and non-nursing) as well as nonprofessional health care providers. Both lines and levels of nursing become types of caring as well (Jarrin 2006). So, practices and practical programs that focus primarily on body-system/disease frameworks can be seen as adequate technical practices, but they are incomplete with respect to professional *Caritas* knowledge-driven practices. Such limited outer-world, right-quadrant practice frameworks are incomplete and inadequate with respect to notions of *Caritas Nursing* and a more mature disciplinary Caring Science context.

If action is informed only by the right-sided quadrant objective field, nursing can be and often is reduced to a task, an end in and of itself. Likewise, the person/patient is reduced to the physical "case," to the moral status of object. As this slippery situation occurs, it allows acts to be performed that are inconsistent with an ethic of caring that honors the "face," the whole person. For example, if another human being is reduced to the moral status of object, one can begin to justify doing things to the other as object, something one would never do to a fully functioning, whole person.

However, if such practices are located within a total-knowledge, energetic, integral chakra system, those same highly technical, concrete tasks (manifest in the outer right-side quadrant/lower chakras) can be informed/transformed by a left-quadrant evolved consciousness and intentionality of the nurse who is working from the left quadrant, with an awareness that the whole is affected. Likewise, even if the starting point is the right quadrant, the *Caritas Nurse* is aware that she or he is affecting the left-quadrant experiences. They are the same.

In a professional, evolved Caring Science/*Caritas Process* model, these basic tasks and body-physical acts are highly regarded, respected, and viewed from a larger lens; they are viewed from the left-side quadrant as well as the evolved energetic chakra system. Thus, the task, basic need, or physical care is not isolated from the whole person, nor is it isolated from the total disciplinary Caring Science knowledge system.

To explore the chakra energetic system in more depth for the *Caritas Nurse*, we seek wisdom traditions and perennial philosophies across time and cultures. Such ancient knowledge, often located within the left quadrant model, instructs us on ancient truths associated with directing our life force and energy source in the outer world.

These chakra energy system understandings and evolution help us understand how we embody and balance our energies of body and soul, of thought and action, of physical and mental, for health and healing. The system of primary energies is both/and, not either/or; it is both physical and spiritual. It develops and guides us throughout life toward an evolving consciousness and wholeness of being, transcending illness and disease. The energetic spiritual-physical chakra system lines up with the left and right quadrant model. Thus, there is room for wholeness of the practitioner and his or her evolution toward becoming more human, more caring, more healing and humane while simultaneously allowing the profession to locate its actions within a whole knowledge system for any practice epistemology (Hagedorn personal communication, 2006).

Our bodies contain an immanent blueprint for healing, in that humans are energy duplicates of a spiritual power, a life energy force connecting us to universal energy, sometimes referred to as the "Divine power system" of the universe (Myss 1996:64). In other words, for every physical aspect of the body and its manifestation on the physical plane, there is a metaphysical overlay of an energetic life force. This perspective gives an entirely different meaning and purpose to understanding how to assist with basic human needs; it incorporates a sacred energetic framework whereby self and others can be helped to co-create their own health and healing while learning to live life more fully. Or this framework can help nurses assist others in more fully mobilizing the energetic life force of self and other through the sacred act of attending to so-called basic human needs.

According to Myss in her 1996 work (my guide for the perspective here), "our biological design is also a spiritual design" (1996:64); thus, energy and spirit come together. It is interesting that this biological-spirit (energy) connection view of humanity and nursing phenomena has been advanced by Nightingale (1969) and Martha Rogers (1970) and explored by others, including Macrae (2001), Newman (1994), Watson (1999, 2005), and Watson and Smith (2002).

Myss (1996) makes these connections more explicit, however, integrating the spiritual-energetic system with the biological-physical, including health challenges, physical and emotional suffering, illness, and diseases. She therefore creates possibilities for understanding that all human stress corresponds to a spiritual (or metaphysical) crisis at some level—thus presenting an opportunity for deeper learning and evolving of one's consciousness (Newman 1994) toward healing/health.

Finding solutions for assisting self and other with basic needs then takes on an entirely different meaning, inviting each person to gain insight regarding his or her own energy system and accessing, redirecting, and balancing one's own spirit/energy/power for reclaiming/ returning to one's original wholeness-of-being.

CHAKRA ENERGY BODY SYSTEM

This revised framework acknowledges the connectedness of each basic need and the holographic nature of all the needs, in that the needs of the whole (person) are contained within each part/each act. The entire caring consciousness embraces each part/each act.

211

The unity of oneness of mind-body-spirit is acknowledged. The physical is overlaid by the metaphysical, the physical with the nonphysical-energetic-spiritual dimensions of our humanity, the sacred with the profane or ordinary.

Within this expanded holographic view, we can acknowledge the reality of basic needs and a way to think about them for intellectual purposes, both as identified separate basic needs for physical survival—commonly the focus of nursing care—and as evolving spirit-filled needs, also needed for soul survival of sorts. Thus, we grasp that each physical need has a metaphysical overlay. Moreover, in a *Caritas Nursing* model we acknowledge that each physical act carries a spirit-

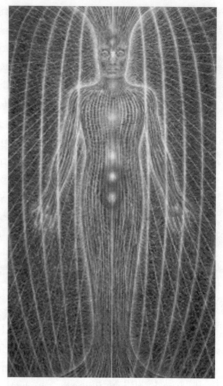

Figure 21. Art by Alex Grey's Sacred Mirrors, *depicting "transpersonal caring."* www.alexgrey.com.

filled energy. We expand and extend our focus toward how we assist others in meeting their basic human needs. We shift to considering the deeper *Caritas Consciousness*—the sacred acts of ministering/administering to others in helping them meet their basic needs, not as parts but ministering to a whole person, a whole knowledge system that is unified and spirit-filled.

**BIOPHYSICAL NEEDS AND
CORRESPONDING ENERGETIC CHAKRA SYSTEM**

The basic biophysical needs are considered the most primitive, instinctual, biological needs for physical survival of the body physical, with involuntary organic responses and requirements: food, drink, elimination, ventilation, and sexual expression. These basic needs are associated with the energetic ancient system of chakras, which include the first through the third chakras.

1. First chakra: base chakra—grounding-connecting with Mother Earth energy for full embodiment; also considered the "root chakra." The first chakra is located at the base of the spine. It is related to grounding, connectedness with the energy of Mother Earth; the spiritual significance is related to the material world. The ancient archetypal "truth" associated with this chakra is the truth of "all is one," in that we acknowledge the interconnectedness of all of life and to one another. We are not separate from each other or from the energy of the whole. We are all part of the family of humanity. This belief is a universal spiritual understanding associated with the base chakra as the foundation for life strength (Myss 1996).

This energetic center encompasses physical body support: the base of the spine, legs, bones, feet, rectum, and immune system. It is associated with one's ability to be-in-the-world, to be connected with the earth plane, and to "stand up" for self. This reflects the ability to provide for life necessities, feeling at home, having a physical family, and enjoying group safety and security connected with social and familial order and law (Myss 1996). This energy represents tribal power as an archetype for group identity, group force, willpower, and group belief systems. It connects us with familial meanings; it reflects our identity, associated with a sense of belonging to a group, a culture, a geographic location (Myss 1996). The energy connection is the foundation of emotional and mental health, stability from within the family unit, and early social experiences.

The primary fears inherent in this energetic location are fear of survival, abandonment by the identified group/family, and loss of physical order. The primary strengths associated with this chakra include family "identity, bonding, honor code and the support and loyalty that give one a sense of safety and connection to the physical world" (Myss 1996:164).

The color associated with this first chakra is red.

The Carative Factor/*Caritas Process* most closely related to this chakra is number 8: provision for a supportive, protective, and corrective environment/safe space, healing space whereby physical-nonphysical aspects are included in basic physical care needs: for example, comfort, dignity, safety, privacy, and so on, for maximizing healing.

2. Second chakra: pelvic chakra—associated with sexuality, creativity, and the birthing of new life, whether as ideas or a biological life force. The second chakra is located in the pelvic area. This energy point is attuned to biological design for procreation, creativity, sexual union, and relationships: from *Eros* to *Philos* to *Agape* connections ranging from marriage to friendship to professional bonds and partnerships to *Agape Love*. The sacred dimension operating here is honoring self and other, acting with integrity in all relationships.

This second chakra is considered the "partnership chakra" and is tied to the power of relationships. Here the energy shifts to discovering relationships that satisfy personal and physical needs (Myss 1996). The location is the lower abdomen to the navel area, including sexual organs, large intestine, lower vertebrae, pelvis, hip area, appendix, and bladder. The area is connected to the need for relationships, sexual-creative expression, and our need for control over the physical environment, including money and other forms of expressivity within our environment.

The second chakra is activated by fear of losing control, losing relationships, losing love, being betrayed, and losing power of the physical body. The primary strengths are related to financial survival, protecting oneself, and the ability to establish partnerships, personal property, and decision making (Myss 1996). This is the energetic site of personal-professional, creative expression, whereby individual talents and one's life force are manifest.

The color associated with the second chakra is orange.

Carative Factors/*Caritas Processes* 6 and 9 are most prominent with respect to the second chakra system: CF/CP 6: systematic use of creative problem solving in the caring process, creative use of self and all ways of knowing to engage in the artistry of caring practices; CF/CP 9: assistance with gratification of basic human needs and expressivity.

3. Third chakra: solar plexus chakra—associated with "gut" feelings, the seat of all emotions, emotional urges, instinctual fight-or-flight responses; this energy center connects with the "stomach, pan-

creas, adrenals, upper intestines, gallbladder, liver and the middle spine, located behind the solar plexus" (Myss 1996:167). According to Myss, this center is related to our personal power, the magnetic core of the personality and ego. It is tied to symbolic and energetic pulls between the external world and internalized self. This is the site where primary fears are held, "such as rejection, criticism, failing to meet one's responsibilities; all fears related to physical appearance, aging, fears others will discover our secrets" (Myss 1996:168). The primary strengths from this energy point are "self-esteem, self-respect, and self-discipline, ambition, the ability to generate action, to handle a crisis, courage to take risks, ethics, strength of character" (Myss 1996:168).

The color associated with the third chakra is yellow.

Carative Factor / Caritas Process 5 is most strongly associated with this energetic field: promotion and acceptance of the expression of positive and negative feelings.

These three lower chakras are associated with basic biophysical needs—elimination, food and fluid, ventilation, sexuality. These basic needs are associated with sources of energy from Mother Earth, energy from earth itself as the ground of our Being.

These needs incorporate intimacy, sensuality, body movement, opening the body energetically for freedom of movement, ventilation, and breath, thus also affecting the ventilation need. The solar plexus is the center for the expression of feelings, emotions, fear, anxiety, resentment—stored emotions with a need for expression, the so-called gut emotions.

I resist categorizing the basic needs into lower biophysical and higher-order needs; however, for study and learning purposes, sometimes one must explore the foundational parts even while holding the whole / hologram as background. All biophysical human needs can be framed holographically as those needs that are foreground and basic for human survival and that are instinctual and organic; however, every basic biophysical need has a metaphysical overlay, reflected by the chakra system.

Regarding these identified biophysical needs, we share them with animals as basic survival instincts. These basic needs are primal, primordial, instinctual, often involuntary, and essential to our humanity.

Within a professional *Caritas Consciousness,* there is an honoring of the embodiment of spirit within each need. Every individual need affects and is part of the whole being of the person, and the person's whole being can be reflected in any one need. While there may be a presenting need, the whole is always present as background to the need presenting itself in a given moment.

For our purposes here, the foreground can be the need for food and fluid, elimination, ventilation, activity, and sexuality. These are the most basic survival needs and those closely aligned with the first three chakras.

These basic survival needs are primarily associated with the first three chakras. But once we move to the fourth chakra, we are evolving toward deeper dimensions of our humanity and our connection with higher spirit-filled awareness, beyond the physical realm.

As we move beyond these most basic survival-instinctual–level needs, we can identify other human needs—also basic but at a different level, beyond physical survival and for survival of the spiritual self, in a way. Other needs beyond the basic survival-instinctual needs are those always present in the human, those influenced by cognition, reflection, emotions, desire, evolving consciousness, self-awareness, will, and so on. Examples include the need for self-love, self-esteem, self-control, self-knowledge, self-caring, self-fulfillment, self-awareness, self-acceptance, self-growth, autonomy, relationships, love, connections, and so forth. The evolved human then moves toward the fourth-level archetypal awareness of the energetic life force source.

HUMAN EVOLUTION—HIGHER-CONSCIOUSNESS ENERGY SYSTEMS

4. Fourth chakra: heart chakra—this energetic point is connected with love, compassion; moving from ego-centered, physical-emotive, fear-motivated human to heart-centered human; open to that which connects one with the greater source of life. Here we are moving from the dominant physical plane to a higher/deeper spiritual awakening of the senses and sensibilities. The heart chakra includes the heart and circulatory system, lungs, shoulders and arms, ribs and breasts, diaphragm, and thymus glands (Myss 1996). It is linked to feelings of forgiveness, hope, and trust as well as love, commitment, and compassion. A closed

heart chakra walls up hatred, resentment, bitterness, grief, anger, self-centeredness, and loneliness (Myss 1996). A heart-centered person moves from a cognitive, rational, head-ego focus toward openness to learning, to seeing other ways of Being-in-the-world. One becomes a person whose heart can hold forgiveness; one develops an open heart filled with loving-kindness, equanimity, and mindfulness; a heart open to the paradox of the ability to hold joy and pain, side by side. As the evolved human opens the heart, he or she can discover wisdom seeking/insight/new sight/new ways of seeing and understanding.

I have heard it said that when one opens the heart chakra, one is opening up all other chakra energy points to allow an energetic flow throughout the whole body. The heart chakra is the center for love, compassion, and companionship and opens access to that which is greater than the self on the physical plane of existence; this opens one to connect with the infinite field of universal Love. This chakra teaches us how to act out of love and compassion and caring, recognizing that the most powerful energy we have is love (Myss 1996).

Myss says that more than any other chakra, the "[f]ourth represents our capacity to 'let go and let God.' With its energy we accept our personal emotional challenges as extensions of a Divine plan, which has as its intent our conscious evolution. By releasing our emotional pain, by letting go of our need to know why things have happened as they have, we reach a state of tranquility. In order to achieve that inner peace, however, we have to embrace the healing energy of forgiveness, and release our lesser need for human self-determined justice" (Myss 1996:197–198).

The primary fears associated with the heart chakra include fear of loneliness, commitment, and "following one's heart"; the fear of an inability to protect oneself emotionally; fear of emotional weakness, betrayal. The loss of heart-centered energy can give rise to jealousy, bitterness, anger, hatred, and an inability to forgive others and self (Myss 1996:198). The primary strengths of this chakra include Love, forgiveness, compassion, dedication, inspiration, hope, trust, and the ability to heal oneself and others. Love in its purest form—unconditional Love—is the substance of the Divine. Our hearts are designed to express beauty, compassion, forgiveness, joy, and love. Love is the fuel of our physical and spiritual bodies. Each lesson in life, at some level, is a lesson in some respect about learning more about love (Myss 1996:198–199).

The color associated with the fourth chakra is green.

This fourth heart chakra is highly associated with Carative Factor/ *Caritas Process* 1: humanistic-altruistic values; practice of loving-kindness and equanimity toward self and other. As the *Caritas Nurse* evolves more fully within the *Caritas Model*, she or he is cultivating this energy point; this chakra makes the greatest contribution toward caring-healing practices. The *Caritas Nurse* is open to a heart-centered consciousness evolution, moving beyond the strictly intellectual, technical, ego-head-centered nurse.

Thus, there is a difference between ordinary nursing and *Caritas Nursing*. The difference lies in the evolution of heart-centered consciousness and working from this evolved awareness, including the fourth chakra and above, to address any lower chakra issues. The first *Caritas Process* of loving-kindness and equanimity contributes to the evolution of *Caritas Nursing* practices. Cultivation of this energetic source is foundational for caring-healing work in the world. When the heart chakra is open, we connect with source.

5. Fifth chakra: "throat chakra"—giving voice to one's life force expression in the world. This center is related to expression through the voice to convey one's heartfelt intentions, bringing voice to action, seeing and knowing through mind and heart and evolving consciousness. The organs associated with this energy anatomy include throat, thyroid, trachea, neck vertebrae, mouth, teeth, gums, esophagus, parathyroid, and hypothalamus (Myss 1996:98). According to Myss, the symbolic challenge of this chakra is to progress through the maturation of will, from the perception that everyone and everything has authority over you to the perception that you have authority over you and making onward progress in realizing/awakening to the fact that true authority comes from aligning yourself with the higher will of God/Godhead. This includes a spiritual surrender of ego control to that which is greater. The primary fears are related to having no authority or power of choice within our own lives and our personal-professional relationships. Then, fearing that we have no authority

within ourselves results in being out of control with money, diet, food, drugs, and similar issues; there is fear of another person's control over our well-being. Finally, we fear the will of God, the greatest struggle for releasing control to a higher source (Myss 1996:220).

The primary strengths of this energetic source are faith, self-knowledge, personal authority, and the capacity to make decisions, to stand in place with one's true self and give authentic expression to one's being-in-the-world. The strength comes from deeply knowing that we have the capacity to keep our word to ourselves and to another/others.

The color associated with the fifth chakra is blue.

The Carative Factors/*Caritas Processes* associated with the throat chakra are numbers 2: faith-hope-helping others sustain a deep belief system; and 4: development of an authentic helping-trusting-caring relationship.

6. Sixth chakra: "the third eye"—evolving consciousness involves our mental and reasoning abilities and reflective skills in evaluating our beliefs and attitudes. This chakra resonates with the energies of our psyches, our consciousness forces. The Eastern literature refers to this chakra as the "'third eye' or spiritual center in which mind and psyche cultivate intuitive sight and wisdom" (Myss 1996:237). Thus, it can also be thought of as the chakra of wisdom, higher consciousness, seeing beyond the ego, and developing insight.

The location of the sixth chakra is the center of the forehead. The challenges here are opening the mind, cultivating an impersonal mind, recognizing "false truths" (Myss 1996:237), becoming self-directed, discriminating between thoughts motivated by Love and strength and those motivated by fear and illusion and control. Ultimately, I consider this chakra to represent evolving consciousness and movement toward a higher/deeper level of awakening to one's highest consciousness, which is Love (Watson 2005). The energy connection with the physical body includes the brain, neurological system, pituitary and pineal glands, as well as the eyes, ears, and nose (Myss 1996:237).

The lessons along the way in relation to evolving consciousness include our ability to become a witness to our own beliefs and states of mind, leading to wisdom, serenity, and inner peace. This encompasses the ability to be still in the midst of threats and chaos, to discern power struggles of illusion versus insight within a greater picture of the divine order of the universe and our connection to it.

The primary fears embodied in this area include an unwillingness to look within, fear of inner exploration, and fear of one's shadow side and its attributes. The challenges include being stuck in predetermined mind-sets and beliefs, fear of releasing illusions of the external world, and an unwillingness to explore one's shadow side with equanimity and forgiveness. The primary strengths include cultivation of deeper self-awareness, insights, wisdom, creativity; higher consciousness for intuitive reasoning; and emotional intelligence: in summary, becoming a more evolved human (Myss 1996).

The color associated with the sixth chakra is amethyst violet.

The Carative Factors/ *Caritas Processes* associated with the sixth "third eye" chakra include numbers 1: humanistic-altruistic value system/practice of loving-kindness and equanimity; and 10: allowing for existential-phenomenological-spiritual dimensions in one's own life, evolution; opening and attending to "mystery," deeper truths behind illusions—"allowing for a miracle."*

7. Seventh chakra: "crown chakra"—spiritual transcendent connector. This energy source is our connection to our spiritual nature, our capacity to bring Spirit into our lives and world. It invites grace, mercy, Love, and surrender to enter our lives, allowing for an intimate relationship with the Divine. This chakra opens us to our quiet, inner soul source for alignment with the universal energy of Cosmic Love (Watson 2005), whereby our inner awareness, awakening, and practices of meditation, prayer, and spiritual sacraments allow us to transcend our ego-physical self. The location for this chakra is the top of the head.

This chakra is considered the entry point for the human life force, which pours endlessly into the human energy system from the greater universe, from the God/Godhead (Myss 1996:265). According to Myss (1996), as depicted in the artwork of Hildegard of Bingen (see Figure 19, Chapter 15), "this life force from the universe nourishes the body, the mind, and the spirit. It distributes itself throughout the physical

---

* From interpretation by Resurrection Health in Chicago.

body and the lower six chakras, connecting the entire physical body to the seventh chakra. The energy of the seventh chakra influences all of the other major body systems: the central nervous system, the muscular system, and the skin" (Myss 1996:265).

The seventh chakra contains the energy that inspires and generates devotion, prophetic thoughts, transcendent ideas, and mystical connections. It is reported that this chakra contains the purest form of the energy of grace and Love; it safeguards our capacity for insights, vision, and intuition beyond ordinary consciousness. It is the mystical realm (Myss 1996:266). It can also be considered as closely aligned with the basic human need for self-actualization, but it goes beyond that to the realm of the Divine, the mystical, opening to infinity.

According to Myss, the primary fears associated with the seventh chakra relate to spiritual issues of the "dark side of the soul": fears of abandonment, loss of identity, and loss of our connection with life and those around us. The primary strengths of this chakra include faith in the presence of the Divine, having faith-hope in that which is greater than self, a divine ordering in one's life and experiences, a profound trust that order is unfolding in the midst of chaos, confusion, crises, fears, and so on. This trust, faith, and strength of spirit help one overcome ordinary human fears, to seek devotion, silence, prayer, and patience to cope with unknowns.

The color associated with the seventh chakra is white.

The seventh chakra is the one that allows nurses and others to be "open to a miracle" for self and other. Thus, the Carative Factors / Caritas Processes most closely associated with this chakra are numbers 1: practice of loving-kindness and equanimity; and 10: opening to spiritual-mysterious and existential dimensions of one's life and death: "allowing for a miracle."

Once nurses and other health and healing practitioners connect with their own energy source and attend to evolving their consciousness to a higher/deeper realm, they open up sources of energy for different aspects of their life force and Being-in-the-world while simultaneously uniting with an infinite source of energy, allowing them to transcend any situation. They are then awakened to a greater sense of self, of community, communion, spiritual evolution, and so on.

CHAPTER EIGHTEEN

The **CARITAS NURSE/CARITAS NURSING** and Chakra Systems

One of the characteristics that distinguishes a *Caritas Nurse* and *Caritas Nursing* from ordinary, routine nursing is where and when the nurse places his or her awareness of the deeper dimensions of the entire human energetic range. For example, it could be posited that a routine nurse, not fully awake, could technically be competent and carry out routine care practices at the basic physical, right quadrant level, but he or she would not be a *Caritas Nurse* or be practicing from *Caritas Consciousness.*

The ordinary nurse is more likely practicing from the ego-mind and operating more from the task-based, outer-world–oriented experience, through the exterior objective quadrant focused more on the lower three chakras. With such a restricted focus, there is little to no awareness of the upward consciousness evolution required for *Caritas Nursing.* There is little to no conscious awareness of or attention to the left-quadrant, nonphysical, energetic dimension of consciousness, intentionality, and so on, that informs the outer world of physical care practices. A *Caritas Nurse* seeks to work with all the chakras, allowing an infusion of energy and awareness to work not only with the lower three chakras but also from the fourth chakra and above, opening to an entire knowledge system and allowing one's evolved consciousness, higher energetic openings, and left-quadrant thinking to inform/transform all levels of practice.

The informed *Caritas Nurse* is one who is intentional, evolving, and awake. The professional *Caritas Nurse* is one who attends to and embraces the lower three chakra systems of the body-physical focus as well as the other energetic systems; this type of *Caritas Nursing* integrates the left-quadrant knowledge system with the outer world of tasks and objective technical care. Therefore, the *Caritas Nurse* is one who engages authentically in her or his own *Caritas Consciousness* evolution, opening access to the life energy source from the left-quadrant knowledge system, which results in concrete caring practices that are both physical and metaphysical in nature.

The *Caritas Nurse* is open to work from the fourth chakra upward to the seventh chakra. This becomes a lifelong journey to bring *Caritas Consciousness* and a more complete knowledge-wisdom system into one's personal-professional practices and life work in caring-healing.

The *Caritas Nurse* and *Caritas Nursing* cultivate and manifest the first foundational *Caritas Process*: loving-kindness and equanimity, meditating on opening the heart to evolve beyond the head-centered, ego-fear, and control mind-set so often prominent in routine, nonreflective, institutional nursing. The *Caritas Nurse* is one who works from the fourth through seventh chakras—heart-throat, third eye, and crown—to inform, embody, and embrace practical, concrete acts of caring grounded in the physical earth plane. The chakra system is an archetypal depiction of individual maturation through seven distinct stages (see Chapter 17). The chakras suggest that we evolve and ascend toward the Divine by mastering the seductive pull that keeps us fixed upon and limited to a focus on the lower, base chakras, the exterior right quadrant, and the outer physical-material world as the supreme but limiting focus of human existence.

Each chakra represents a spiritual life lesson or challenge common to all humans. As a person evolves by giving more attention to the deeper/higher aspects of life, she or he gains self-knowledge, wisdom, and true power—all of which are integrated into spirit and the path of spiritual consciousness. Thus, the *Caritas Nurse* is one who enters the path of awakening and moving along this higher path for self while honoring and supporting the journey for others.

CHAKRA SUMMARY

First chakra: lessons related to material-physical world

Second-third chakras: lessons related to sexuality, work, physical desire, material possessions; lessons related to personal, emotional, ego-driven personality and self-esteem

Fourth chakra: lessons related to love, forgiveness, compassion, kindness, equanimity

Fifth chakra: lessons related to giving authentic expression, bringing unique voice to bear upon life choices, will, and one's being with self and other

Sixth chakra: lessons related to open mind, intuition, insights, vision, wisdom, surrender to greater source from the universe

Seventh chakra: lessons related to access to greater source from infinite cosmos; related to one's opening to the highest spiritual source for consciousness evolution.

The *Caritas Nurse* is one who holds a high ethical-spiritual standard of excellence for personal-professional lessons, growth, and Being-in-the-world; one who awakens to his or her spiritual chakra archetypal evolution to deepen the individual's humanity. The *Caritas Nurse* is one who works to ground self in the first three chakras to connect with the energy of planet Earth. The challenge is also to work on opening the fourth chakra and above to evolve as a more mature, civil, moral human being, connecting with the deeper level of Divine nature. Such personal-professional growth and lessons of caring-healing are necessary for *Caritas Nursing* while honoring the basic needs emanating from chakras one, two, and three. Thus, the *Caritas Nurse* engages in cultivating compassionate human caring, working from an open, intelligent heart and mind and spirit-filled consciousness of loving-kindness, equanimity, forgiveness, and compassion for self and other. The *Caritas Nurse* is open to learning lessons from the left knowledge quadrant and the full chakra system as other ways of knowing and evolving, thus opening to honoring one's full self-evolution as well as the fullness of the other, drawing upon an entire knowledge system and a life path for personal/professional evolution. Thus, the *Caritas Processes* within the Philosophy and Science of Caring guide the nurse and the evolved profession and discipline of nursing along the ethical and moral journey and heritage of *Caritas* practices by learning to live the formal theoretical *Caritas Processes* in one's work and world.

This line of thinking allows the *Caritas Nurse* to cultivate the awareness that any physical condition has a metaphysical-energetic mirror at the nonphysical level. Any outer-world, right-quadrant phenomenon has a left-quadrant meaning informing it. Therefore, living, dying, caring-healing health phenomena are multilayered and complex; they are ultimately incapable of being fully known; they are ineffable, reminding us that ultimately we dwell within the mystery of Infinity.

PART V

*Health, Healing, Humanity, and
Heart-Centered Knowing for* Caritas Nursing

Over a century ago, Florence Nightingale established nursing's focus within a context of health and wholeness that contained yet transcended body-physical, limited approaches to health and healing; thus, she embraced the human spirit and nonphysical phenomena that reside within as well as without. She advocated that nursing focus on health and human experiences that affect all humanity across time and space, all ages, nationalities, races, and varieties of human circumstances that we share. Such a focus transcends disease and illness while still accommodating those realities of nursing.

Within the context of *Caritas Nursing,* it can be made more explicit that health and healing notions related to caring are distinctly different from exclusive medical, clinical, body-physical approaches. In this model, health cannot be and is not defined from the standpoint of clinical disease or illness. In this model, health is first and foremost an illusive, if not philosophical, concept and thus has to be individually defined. It is a subjective, inner-life world experience and phenomenon that cannot necessarily be defined by external criteria alone.

Neither health nor illness/disease is an absolute state; rather, they constitute a process of living, growing, evolving, being, experiencing, and learning along life's journey.

Nursing models and theories, from Nightingale onward, have made explicit that health is not simply the absence of disease; they have incorporated many life force dimensions, patterns, and processes related to individual, community, and cultural worldviews. However, the dominant mind-set continues to place both emphasis and dollars on disease rather than on health. Modern, contemporary, sophisticated medical systems still concentrate on sick care rather than well care, prevention, and the quality of living, dying, being, becoming, and so on. Ironically, to compound the issue, most of the health-illness problems that occur most frequently and affect the largest number of people are linked not to specific diseases but rather to psychosocial, lifestyle, social, and environmental conditions and life circumstances.

The confusion of health and healing with medical disease and treatment-cure has generated even more dilemmas, in that medicalized views of humans and the human condition have gradually emerged whereby almost any human experience or condition of living has a medical treatment and a diagnosis affixed to it. The result: a medicalized-clinical approach to life through the increased use of drugs, pharmaceutical-technical interventions, and medical specialization, now almost mandated to deal with life itself.

On the other hand, there is a spiritual emergence and a trend toward a spiritualization of health and illness beyond the limited medicalized views of health, disease, and illness. In this emerging framework, new space is opening for an evolving consciousness for nursing and patients/health care systems alike. There are metaphorical views of disease as an invitation to understand, to gain new meaning for one's life pattern, to see health and illness as evolving consciousness and opportunities for healing—to feel/be more whole, to be-in-right-relation, to experience more unity of mind-body-spirit regardless of external conditions, circumstances, physical limitations, and so on.

Thus, the emerging models no longer adhere to a conventional "physicalistic" orientation to health, to illness, to life, to death.

Health and wholeness and illness and disease can operate simultaneously. Each can be experienced as an opportunity to return home to one's core essence and center, to what is most important for one's being and learning through the illness, to gain energy and balance from one's source and inner center, to return/repattern to the healing and wholeness awaiting as a vibrating possibility for self/other, open to unknowns, the mystery, the miracles.

Within this emerging awareness of a deeper, more meaningful approach to life and healing and wholeness, beyond disease per se, nursing and health care professionals are challenged from within and without to respond to a higher/deeper dimension of caring and healing that draws upon the richest sources of their own humanity. Thus, nursing is experiencing a crossroads of awakening to a new order for a new era of human health history. Nurses are now challenged to bring their full self, their human presence of caring and healing, into moments with others. Nurses in this model of *Caritas Nursing* are invited and expected to engage in self-care practices that elevate their consciousness, that open their hearts and higher chakra fields of energy whereby they realize that they are the field, they are the environment, they are affecting the entire energetic field that radiates out to the larger universe, they are affecting the totality of health care. The universal, infinite field of energy of Cosmic Love (Levinas 1969) and nursing's access to this field for self and other have profound implications for the future of nursing and human health care worldwide.

CHAPTER NINETEEN

Human Experiences: Health, Healing,
and **CARITAS NURSING***

It seems to me that one of the reasons we have been limited and restricted in our evolution, in the ways we have defined ourselves, our jobs, and our science is because we have failed to see that work in the field of caring-healing intersects with the very tasks of not only "facing our humanity," but deepening our humanity. Indeed, the very endeavors we are embarked upon with respect to being human are the very endeavors we mirror, reflect, and engage in as part of our caring-healing work with self and other. Just what are these human tasks that intersect with the Caring Science model? Well, the four tasks include the essential human tasks for healing and deepening our humanity:

---

* Excerpts: Reprinted with permission from J. Watson (2005). *Caring Science as Sacred Science*. Philadelphia: F. A. Davis, 132–139.

Forgiveness; Offering Gratitude; Surrendering and Overcoming Fear and Pride.

There are at least four or five other more abstract human endeavors we all share in our collective humanity. These transcend our common work, regardless of professional/personal background. We learn these practices through love and authentic engagement, acknowledgement of self and other, of offering gratitude, forgiveness, validation and recognition to self and others. As we cultivate these shared human tasks, we establish a foundation for a Caritas consciousness, helping to overcome fear, anger, competition, jealousy, defensiveness and so on, opening to beneficial emotions and higher/deeper consciousness for love and joy, healing emotions and trust in life.

As we engage in these practices, we become more honest with our self, more able to surrender to what is/to love what is, rather than fighting it.

We can request and offer forgiveness and blessings from self and those we may have hurt. In this way we learn to bless and forgive persons, situations and circumstances that otherwise would immobilize and freeze us in our emotions. These simple yet profound human acts help us overcome fear and pride that separate us from our true nature and our connection with all that is, human and universal.

We may not even be aware that these are the tasks toward developing a mature wise heart, until they are brought to our conscious attention and awareness. These endeavors include at least the following challenges for locating our work, our science, and our human evolution within Caring Science (Watson 2003):

- Healing our relationship with Self and Others/Planet Earth/Universe

- Understanding and transforming our own and other's suffering

- Deepening and expanding our understanding of living and dying; acknowledging the shadow-light cycle of the great sacred circle of life

- Preparing for our own death.

HEALING OUR RELATIONSHIP WITH
SELF/OTHER/PLANET EARTH/UNIVERSE

Within this framework, we now realize, more than ever, that before we can engage in healing practices, including medical and nursing practice, we have to deal with healing our relationship with self and Other, in that it all begins with self and radiates out to the universe. Within the field of health care, and nursing in particular, there is a long history of being unkind, if not cruel among ourselves; likewise, there are stories and research studies that condemn medical education and authoritarian practices that perpetuate unkind, cruel, and in some instances, abusive practices in health professional education and practice field. Yet, we are charged with moral and social expectations to *care* and to be *healers*.

This focus on healing our relationships becomes very personal, yet it affects, if not informs, our professional practices. This basic task of being human and becoming more humane intersects with our professional focus in caring-healing. We forget that our health care work is greater than we have acknowledged; the human nature of our work has been too small and limited in its scope in relation to the rich, complex nature of this deeply human work.

To engage in healing our self and our relationship with each other and beyond, the practices of *Forgiveness, Offering Gratitude, and Surrendering* to higher/deeper source for consolation, creativity, insight and heart-centered action, is a way to begin. It seems that our relationship with our self is most critical to all other aspects of healing work, including our own personal health. It starts with self and moves in concentric radiating circles out to all whom we touch physically, locally, non-locally, and energetically. We return again and again to these basic human practices to stay alive, awake, and to sustain our humanity. As Rumi put it:

> It doesn't matter that you've broken
> your vow a thousand times, still
> come, and yet again, come.

AND his reminder/rejoinder for our living/Being/Becoming:

Don't pretend to know
something you haven't experienced.
There's a necessary dying. . . .
Be ground. Be crumbled, so wildflowers will come up
where you are. You've been
stony for too many years. Try something different. Surrender.

JALALUDDIN RUMI

BETTERING OUR UNDERSTANDING OF HUMAN SUFFERING: HELPING TO TRANSFORM ITS MEANING

It is widely held that to be human is to suffer. All major religions and wisdom traditions and text deal with suffering in one way or another. One of our human tasks at the individual and collective level[s] is to make meaning of our own suffering. We take it from the abstract concept into our daily lives, when and where we are actually witnessing and experiencing our own and others' real, overt suffering.

However, we also know from our human experiences that we can find new meanings and we seek meaning to assist us when we are most vulnerable, fearful, and "suffering" the slings and arrows known as life. It seems we learn through the deeply personal encounters with suffering that we learn we can't go around life, we have to go through the experience in order to not only survive, but to thrive, to sustain a sense of hope for continued existence, living.

We also are informed both by our experiences and testing of how to live, as well as by our sacred texts for how to live, that as long as we adhere to a fixed, solid, physical dimension as all there is to life, then we are locked into concrete psyche and physical pain. Tolle (1999), in his contemporary writings as well as ancient Buddhist texts, reminds us that all suffering is ego-centered and due to resistance. For example, the Buddhist's basic philosophy was considered with inner transformation by achieving insight into the "Four Noble Truths" of Buddhism (Solomon and Higgins 1997:19):

1. Life is suffering.

2. Suffering arises from selfish craving.

3. Selfish craving can be eliminated.

4. One can eliminate selfish craving by following the right way.

The right way to liberation, enlightenment, or elimination / transformation of suffering is called the *Eightfold path* of Buddhism which consists of (1) right seeing; (2) right thinking; (3) right speech; (4) right action; (5) right effort; (6) right living; (7) right mindfulness; and (8) right meditation (Solomon and Higgins [1997]:19).

These are big orders for how to live a life that is full of suffering due to impermanence, when we cling for permanence and delude ourselves that there is a permanent self and permanency of life. At another level, the suffering is a result of our craving for separateness, for our individuality, our independence, separating and distancing ourselves from each other, other human beings, as well as our environment, our world, our universe. This too contributes to human suffering according to contemporary science as well as ancient sacred texts.

This underlying reality of impermanence is tied up with our avoidance of participating in the cyclical nature of all of life and to the law of impermanence of all things. That is, underneath what is perceived as fixed and unchanging reveals itself as a living paradox, a yin-yang, *both-and* phenomenon. Underneath the felt suffering and pain, there resides an abiding presence, the infinity of universal Love as a field that offers an abiding peace, an unchanging deep stillness, an uncaused joy that transcends good and bad, pain and no-pain (Tolle 1999). This underneath abiding field that holds us in the midst of the constant movement is what T. S. Eliot named *"the still point."*

At the big picture level, this impermanence cycle mirrors the great circle of birth-death; creation-destruction, growth-dissolution, manifest-unmanifest fields. In this way of understanding change and impermanence, everything is rising up and falling away; expanding and contracting, mirroring the breath and rhythm of life's natural energetic processes in all things.

Buddha made this discovery the very heart of his teaching: the cyclical nature and impermanence of the universe. Everything is in constant flux. Our challenge to find new understanding about the nature of human suffering is not only all of our human tasks; it is a professional task in that for a caring-healing practitioner / scientist the two intersect. And as we seek new understandings that deepen our humanity, we become more humane, compassionate, wise and healing in our work and world. Our task as health and caring-healing professionals is to realize that in both our science worlds, as well as our practice world, our work and jobs have been too narrow for the deep human nature of the work that we really are confronted with in our caring-healing relationships with self, others and our universe. A reality to live is to find the still point in the midst of the law of constant change; to find the abiding peace and presence of divine intelligence, a universal field of Love that transcends all the felt change that we solidify and freeze in our experience, contributing to more pain, more suffering. But in the deeper / wisdom understanding and experiencing that can take us *beyond-suffering*, we suddenly realize that there is a marked difference between pain with suffering and pain without suffering. It is how we perceive and allow the impermanence to move through us, not clinging, freezing, and fixing the temporary condition or circumstance in our mind, our bodies, emotions, or even our hearts.

In the end, we are always "in training" and if and when we practice this understanding and acceptance of suffering, we learn to transform that suffering into hope, love and deep compassion (Thich Nhat Hanh 2003). As Thich Nhat Hanh reminds us, the foundation of hope, love, and compassion is already there in our hearts and minds, awaiting our entering this new place of consciousness and learning to dwell there, thus transforming suffering into a deeper level of living.

SUFFERING

One way is to grasp the reality of suffering and learn at a personal level how new insights can change our views, if not transform our views of life. This change happened to me at a personal experiential level when I had my eye injury and was experiencing acute and unbearable pain at the time. I learned the difference between having pain *with* suffering and having pain *without* suffering. I learned this through the practice of deep meditation whereby I was able to witness my pain and watch it as a continuous movement-of-energy, rising up and falling away; it was when I resisted the pain and solidified or fixed it that it congealed, so to speak, and became more painful and brought more suffering, both physically and emotionally. So, at a physical level of

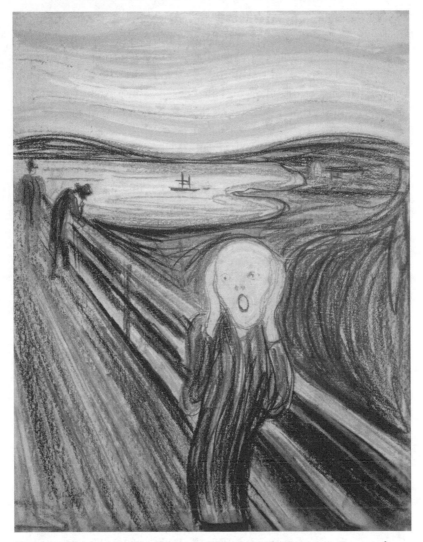

Figure 22. Geschrei, *by Edvard Munch. Collection, Oslo Kommunes Kunstsamlinger, Munch-Museet.*

experience, I learned to meditate my way through a great deal of the pain, or at least catch myself when I was resisting. In opening myself to the experience itself, as a witness of my own experience, the pain passed through me energetically, in waves of energy, expanding and contracting. It was the contracting and congealing that brought the most suffering, but by watching it move beyond, and through, me; by staying still with the process, it became some sort of a miracle. That is only one small example of physical pain, but the same process can be explored and discovered for life itself, as well as other forms of pain, be they psychic, emotional, mental. These become part of our entire journey toward greater health and healing/wholeness of being.

DEEPENING AND EXPANDING OUR UNDERSTANDING OF LIVING AND DYING: ACKNOWLEDGING THE SHADOW/LIGHT CYCLE OF THE GREAT SACRED CIRCLE OF LIFE

While we adhere to health and curing/caring and healing as our primary mission in this health care work, we also now have to acknowledge that we work within the great circle of life-death. This reality recognizes that we all share this common task of facing our humanity at a deep level, both personally and professionally. What we do is not without consequences, in that one way or another we are contributing to and co-participating within the web of life. In all of our work and actions we are working within the universal energy field of infinity that enfolds and surrounds and upholds all of life—time, past, present, future; time before and time after the earth plane of existence; spirit transcending physical body transcending death as we know it. So, making-meaning, and seeking-meaning about understandings of life and living and dying; deepening our view and appreciation for all of life is part of our human quest. David Bohm proposed that *meaning is a form of Being* (Weber 1986:18); that is, it is realizing that through our meanings we change nature's being. Humans' meaning-making capacity turns us into nature's partner in shaping our evolution. Bohm suggests that what we are actually doing by engaging in dialogue with the cosmos is changing its idea of itself (Weber 1986). This perspective is quite awesome and humbling to consider the majesty of the universe and our relationship with it in a deeper way.

Renee Weber believes this deeper diminution is activated in all the participants through dialogue whereby our own world-line/song-line intersects with and forms part of the process. This song-line of relationship and intersecting web of life "continues and carries over from the cosmos into our own spiritual journey" (Weber 1986:18).

Part of this meaning-making quest for a greater depth of life-death and our place within it is related to an awakening: awakening to the fact that we are Spirit made whole in physical manifestation. As Teilhard de Chardin noted, we are not just physical beings having a spiritual experience; rather we are spiritual beings having a physical experience. This perspective now converges with language such as manifest and non-manifest field of existence. This view of awakening seeks to honor the unknown, the unseen as much as the seen, often realizing the illusion of what we think we know and see of the physical plane to not be true reality. Just as in exploring deeper dimensions of suffering, we learn that what we perceive as suffering, at one level, is our own congealing and freezing of the divine flow of life energy; in other words, not being in flow with natural laws of nature and natural timeless rhythm of all things in the universe; the seasons, the tides, the cycles of time and existence; the coming-into-being of living creatures and the passing-out-of-being on physical plane existence, be it human or other living things. Everything is constantly changing and deepening our understanding of this mystery of life, coming and going in our midst, including our own.

PREPARING FOR OUR OWN DEATH

When you see and accept the impermanent nature of all life forms,
A strange sense of peace comes upon you.

TOLLE (2003:105)

Another final human task we all share, which intersects with the nature of caring-healing work, is coming face-to-face in preparing for our own death. As the sages say, without honoring death, we are not fully alive. Indeed, in the cosmic sense again, we are dying every moment, in that with each breath we experience the miracle of life and the precious, yet delicate, nature of how we are held in the hands of that which is greater than us. And at a deeper metaphysical or metaphorical level or within Native American cosmology or any indigenous belief system, death is not the end, it is a continuation of the sacred wheel of life. And as the expression goes: Who is to say that life is not death, and death is not life. And we certainly glimpse situations in which we are called to ask about the living dead we sometimes feel in our hearts and/or in our midst. In preparing for our death, we learn from those who are our teachers along the way. Those who are undergoing the life-death transition can be a gift for our learning and preparation. They can teach us if we listen and are able to be present to their experience and be there with and for them as we are able.

When working with others during times of despair, vulnerability and unknowns, we are challenged to learn again, to re-examine our own meaning of life and death. As we do so, we engage in more authentic processes and practices to cultivate and sustain caring-healing for self and others. Such care and practices elicit and call upon profound wisdom and understanding, beyond knowledge, that touch and draw upon the human heart and soul. However, this learning can be informed by our science, a science that honors the whole. A Science of Caring that opens to the infinity of our learning and evolving. Death is thus not a medical anomaly or the most horrible of all events as our culture has us believe, but as Tolle reminds us, the most natural thing in the world. "There is not anything that is not subject to birth and death; there is not anything on the earth plane that is eternal" (Tolle 2003:109).

In this reminder of heart-centered knowing and wisdom beyond words and conventional knowledge, our basic humanness transcends circumstances, time, and place. Our being and becoming more humane and evolved allows us to engage once again in compassionate human service and science, motivated by love, both human and Cosmic. From this place of deepening our humanity, we offer to our self, and those whom we meet on our path, our compassionate response for fulfilling our chosen life's work and calling. In encountering and facing death of self and others, we are in sacred space, touching the mystery of life itself, dwelling in the space of Infinity.

Just as it is in our personal lives during crises or illness, tragedy, loss, or impending death we ponder spiritual questions that go beyond the physical material world, it is here in our evolving professional-scientific life that we may need to ponder new meaning. In our conventional dispirited, physical-technical life form, deathbed of sorts, Caring Science offers new freedom, new space to reconsider a deeper meaning of caring-healing work and phenomena.

It is here in our wounded, broken science models that a Caring Science may reorient us or, at least, point us toward another science model that may be more hopeful for understanding and living our caring and healing. It is here, in this transition, this space and place between the breaths, that we can quiet the pace, bow down, and take in new energy and new directions to inspire (inspirit-ensoul) our work and our world. The more science learns, it seems the greater nature and life's mystery grow. As we seek to increase our knowledge and wisdom of our deepening and expanding humanity, it opens science to even more profound beauty and wonder of life's infinite cosmic connectedness and oneness in which we reside (Weber 1986).

So, within Caring Science, we now have a new call to bring us back to that which already resides deep within us and intersects with the focus of caring and healing at this time. It allows us to uncover the latent infinite Love in our work and world and connect with contemporary philosophies that invite Love and Caring through our ethics of Being-Becoming-Belonging. This revised text invites us to make the leap of faith back into metaphysics and a moral foundation for our science and our life, to incorporate into our science the reverence for the sacredness of life and death and our shared human heart-centered evolution.

Ultimately and finally, may we be inspired with a renewed commitment to *remember* who we are and why we came here: *To Love, To Serve and To Remember* (Astin 1991).

PART VI

Critiquing Nursing Education

CHAPTER TWENTY

CARITAS CURRICULUM and *Teaching-Learning**

BRINGING THE HEART AND
MIND TOGETHER FOR *CARITAS* EDUCATION*

This chapter extends the concept of *Caritas* teaching and learning to nursing education. It explores the nature of professional nursing and health-sciences education and curricula from a moral, philosophical framework of *Caritas* thinking, encompassing an expanded view of nursing as a human-caring science. Contemporary theories and philosophies of caring and healing and their relevance to nursing and health-sciences education are integrated in the framework. A focus on educating students for a values-based practice morally guided to create reflective, humane *Caritas* practitioners is explored, along

---

* With special acknowledgment to John Drummond for reviewing and offer
ing editorial suggestions for this chapter.

245

with current and futuristic pedagogies directed toward transformative teaching and learning. Previous works in nursing education that underpin this perspective are integrated into a contemporary framework that offers both a moral and a scientific model for considering caring as an ethic, an ontology, an epistemic and praxis endeavor, as well as an educational/pedagogical challenge.

> To take love seriously
> and to bear and to learn it like a task,
> this is what people need.
> For one human being to love another,
> that is perhaps the most difficult of all our tasks,
> the ultimate, the last test and proof,
> the work for which all other work
> is but a preparation.
>
> RAINER MARIA RILKE

One of the greatest disappointments in modern times has been an exclusive focus on the head and the mind, on rational, cognitive thinking as the basis for teaching-learning, almost to the exclusion of the heart and emotions. As a caring profession, where are we to learn the ultimate, the last test and proof of the work of humanity with which we deal: Human Caring/*Caritas*/Love?

Within a critique of knowledge and education, curriculum and learning, we have a new awareness, an awakening to the fact that every epistemology becomes an ethic (Palmer 2004). A fundamental conflict has prevailed within our institutions of higher learning that has already caught up with us in the Western world of science and professionalism. Everything has consequences. The types and ways of teaching and learning that have prevailed at the cognitive, intellectual, rational level alone are formative to our human development; they are shaping the lives of human beings and forming, informing, or deforming our mind-sets and actions as people and as professionals.

As Palmer (2004:2) profoundly asked, "What ethical formation and deformation has this approach to education created in our lives?" suggesting overtly a relationship between our knowledge and violence: the violence of knowledge (and language of power, control, domination, superiority). This form of knowledge development as often practiced in institutions of higher learning has "lent itself to subtle and pervasive forms of violence," to our personal, social, and professional ontological being, our epistemology informing our ethics, our human mode of living (2004:2).

By "violence," Palmer means more subtle forms than dropping a bomb or hitting someone physically. Rather, he refers to violence associated with "violating the integrity" of the other, whether the other is the earth, another human being, or another culture. This mode of learning and knowledge is tied up with the Western academy emphasis on three dominant ways of thinking, teaching, and learning, which according to Palmer (2004) are intended to guide our professional and personal lives: "objective, analytic, and experimental."

Each of these three dominant ways of learning, of valuing, of teaching, of knowing is critiqued by Palmer in his classic paper presented at the 2004 USA Fetzer Institute–sponsored conference, "21st Century Learning Initiatives." He points out the misguided myth that one cannot know anything truly well unless it is held at arm's length, at a distance, at great remove from self—thus perpetuating a chasm between the knower and the known. This myth reinforces the belief that knowledge is tainted, distorted, and untrustworthy if close to the individual; thus, one cannot possibly generate valid knowledge from a personal connection with the data or information.

OBJECTIVISM AS MYTHIC EPISTEMOLOGY—EPISTEMOLOGY-AS-ETHIC

Within this mythic epistemological system of knowledge, of learning, of valuing, of teaching as objective, Palmer reminds us that we create a profound fear of subjectivity, a fear of relatedness, of entering into a relationship with that which we know. Using the metaphors of the Gulf War and the Vietnam War, he points out different explanations of the approaches related to objectivity and subjectivity. For example, the Gulf War, in which tens of thousands of noncombatants were murdered, was a largely acceptable war to the majority of the American public because it was fought from a distance, detached and removed, because it was an air war conducted at arm's length through the miracles of electronics and engineering and new technology. Thus, he noted, the Gulf War had overcome the "Vietnam syndrome," which was a subjective war, fought face-to-face, a war that tore us apart because we were so troubled by the subjective evidence. This contrast of these past wars and their effect on the public worldwide also helps to explain in part the growing resistance to the Iraq War, which is closer and closer to the day-to-day world of the public around the world.

With this line of thinking, one can begin to see how our thin line of epistemology crosses over into ethics. That is how objectivity for its own sake and the mythology of rightness create cruelty if they do not accurately portray how events/knowledge really exist in the world.

The objectivist mythology, whether in war metaphors or personal life events, is a distortion of both reality and knowledge, a distortion of values; it is a distortion of science and how science is done. Palmer helps us remember: great knowing and great learning are not simply done objectively. Paradoxically, they constitute a dance between the objective and subjective, between intimacy and distance, between the personal, inner-life world and the outer, professional-political domain. This is true in all disciplines, not just nursing. The mythology of objectivism is "more about [power] and control over the world, or over each other [or a given phenomenon], more a mythology of power than a real epistemology that reflects how real knowing proceeds." As such, perpetuating this mythology of objectivism does not help us to see that "every epistemology becomes an ethic" (Palmer 2004:2) and affects how we value and see the different phenomena in our world.

NIGHTINGALE AS EXEMPLAR OF UNDERSTANDING "EPISTEMOLOGY AS ETHIC"

The story of Nightingale and her hands-on approach to knowing is a historic as well as a modern example of the "dance" of great knowing, the paradoxical integration of the subjective and objective. She skillfully wove together objective data and subjective visions, a personal sense of calling for her mission and outer-world life's work that transcended any objectivist logic of her era. Yet her internal ethics guided her approach to knowing, to valuing, to teaching, and to learning. She is arguably an exemplar of living the paradox of oneness with her being, knowing, doing in the world. This is not to say that we must agree with everything she said and did, but it is worth remembering that her weltanschauung (worldview) was largely what motivated her actions as one of the key figures in the emergence of modern nursing.

THE ANALYTIC AND EXPERIMENTAL AS MYTHIC EPISTEMOLOGY

Just as objectivism is a mythology yet can destructively become our ethic, ethos, and mind-set for teaching, learning, scholarship, and so on, Parker Palmer pointed out the same misstep with the notion that "analytic" and "experimental" mean "Being scientific." Analytic, as he makes explicit, means that once you have objectified a phenomenon as something to be studied, you are then free to cut it into little pieces to see how it works; to break it down into parts, hold it at a distance, analyze it, and thus understand it. Palmer used this cutting-things-up phenomenon in order to look at, to understand, something "objectively," as a metaphor for what education often does to the human mind and human heart and human soul—the human experience in its totality. Palmer argues that this great facility for taking things apart, dissecting them to the point that one cannot know the original, is a form of violence in that it cultivates a lack of sensitivity and little capacity for putting things back together, including the human heart.

The same is true for the myth of "experimental," in that the mythology of objectivity, analytic, sets up mythological imprints that suggest that once things are objectified, dissected into parts, we are free to experiment. This focus in turn leads us to justify reducing a human to the moral status of object so we can objectively know, study, experiment, and conduct science.

This form of experimentation with humans and nature leads us to seek designs with what we think the world should be like, to control and dominate the outcome, so to speak, with our logic, our distant data, and our moving things around from their original form. We do this without paying attention to potentially destructive outcomes for self, society, humanity, the environment, and nature alike. This thesis of Palmer's about the epistemological myths that deform our ethics reminds me of the rhetorical and haunting question a physician asked me during my first trip to mainland China in the late 1970s: "Why do Americans and Canadians always ask about the parts but never about the wholes?" Of course, his question does not apply to everyone universally, but it lingers.

PARTS AND WHOLES: THE RHETORICAL AND HAUNTING QUESTIONS FOR NURSING EDUCATION

This rhetorical question about parts and wholes should perhaps continue to linger in our minds. With our dominant mythologies of knowledge, teaching, valuing, learning, and being that focus on parts while we are challenged to work with wholes and whole human beings and whole knowledge systems, there is an argument for wondering, are we to remain helpless and even destructive to ourselves and to our knowledge of human caring, healing, health, and humanity if we fail to ask and address the other side of the epistemological mythology? We have new questions we are ethically challenged to address, especially for professional nursing education and *Caritas* curricula and Caring pedagogy:

- How do we put the parts back into the whole?
- How do we integrate facts with meanings?
- How do we acknowledge that the personal is also the professional?
- How do we allow our ethics to become our epistemology rather than perpetuating epistemological myths that deform our ethics?
- How do we honor ontology-of-relationship and caring relationship as ethic, as epistemology, as pedagogy and praxis for advancing professional nursing?
- How do we create, develop, and practice Caring Science rather than the dominant biomedical-technological science model?
- How do we integrate, honor, and sustain humanity and relational *Caritas* in the midst of technological advances?
- How do we create a *Caritas* curriculum and *Caritas Nurses* for twenty-first-century nursing and healing health care?

ADDRESSING THE RHETORICAL EDUCATIONAL
QUESTIONS AND ISSUES FOR THE TWENTY-FIRST CENTURY

Today, we are facing these critical questions about the consequences of our teaching-learning models. There is a worldwide search for more than status quo approaches to education and knowing, whereby there are also efforts to avoid the divided self mind-set with its violent repercussions.

Native Americans and indigenous cultures around the globe offer insights and wisdom beyond our extant mythic epistemology. Their whole-worldview approach to knowing is by honoring human life within the context of a comprehensive cosmology that informs views of life and death, living and dying, and humans' place in the universe. In their cosmology, life and death, knowledge, and all of life's events are one great circle of the web of life. Real life, health, and illness stories of healing, survival, changing, dying are beyond humans' full control; they have to be considered within the web of life itself, from a wiser knowledge system, a larger cosmology, a larger ethic than our human lens. This shift to a larger cosmology is essential if we are to sustain humanity for both human and planetary survival at this point in history (Levinas 1969).

RECONSIDERING NIGHTINGALE AS EXEMPLAR AND MODEL

Florence Nightingale, the founder of modern nursing, was a visionary with respect to cosmologies of wholeness, expanded epistemologies, and foundational ethics and values that guided her in her work and her world. She possessed insights, wisdom, intuition, vision, and knowledge that incorporated entire knowledge systems. Yet the rhetorical and realistic questions and issues triggered by the Chinese physician in 1978 are still facing nursing education and health-sciences education today.

Nightingale's vision and focus for nursing and health serve us all, once again, as an exemplar as we consider and reconsider these haunting questions for nursing education's future. For example, she perceived people as multidimensional beings, with all aspects addressed by medicine and nursing. Her views of health incorporated physical, psychological, mental, and social, as well as environmental and spiritual, feelings, intellect, and relationships. Nightingale stated (quoted in Dossey, Keegan, and Guzzetta 2005:103) that health "is not only to be well, but to be able to use every power we have to use." Her ethics and values guided her approach to learning and practicing. Dossey and colleagues (2005:54) pointed out that Nightingale's recurring message was about what constituted the "lifelong journey of healing and what is required to understand the wholeness of human existence. To her, healing was the blending of the nurse's inner life with her outer life to facilitate her creative expression of love." This process was one of inner peace radiating from the nurse to the person receiving care so the person would feel safe and in harmony. Such a perspective was one of the authenticity and unconditional human presence of the nurse and engagement in "self-reflection, and connections with the Divine" (Dossey, Keegan, and Guzzetta 2005:54).

In Nightingale's framework for healing and health, kindness, caring, and compassion were part of the unifying process, the "interconnectedness with self, others, nature, and God/Life Force/Absolute/Transcendent" (Dossey, Keegan, and Guzzetta 2005:54). Nightingale's vision and advice for nursing education and practice have relevance today as they did in history, in that they pointed toward timeless dimensions of nursing, learning, teaching, and clinical care that still need attention.

Nightingale's vision pointed to the need to put the parts back into the whole, to create space whereby a reunion can occur between physical and metaphysical. The rest of this chapter seeks to address these timeless yet pressing issues within the context of a value-based nursing education. By overcoming the mythology of epistemology as stagnant, deforming, and detached, a living ethic, epistemology, and ontology of wholeness, relationship, and human caring-healing will be developed. Such a values-guided epistemology is built on a moral, philosophical Caring Science model for education, for curriculum, for teaching and learning that allows *Caritas Nursing* to evolve.

CARING SCIENCE AS CONTEXT FOR NURSING EDUCATION

As a reminder, the term *Caritas* has the Latin meaning of care or a certain form of love. This differentiates it from love as *amore*. The latter tends to be a love in which self-interest is involved, whereas *Caritas* denotes a caring or love for something that lies beyond the self-interest of any given individual. Further, *Caritas* is not intended to convey a mere sentiment. The term suggests a certain form of care, a care to be cognizant of the other. This notion is related to the Greek word *agape*, meaning literally "open" or "attitude of wonder" but in this case "open to the other," to the *difference* of other. Levinas develops this point by using the image of "the face" to distinguish the difference of other, this particular individual who differs from a universal other—an "other" that tends toward the impersonal or impartial in which the face is largely marginalized because it is unseen.

For the moment, we can say that Caring Science is a model of thought and practice in which biomedical science and technical evidence alone are not simply blended with *Caritas* but that biomedical science and evidence per se are subsumed within an ethical dimension as the prime consideration—that which recognizes "the face," beyond "any case."

In this respect, "Caring Science" can be defined as "an evolving ethical-epistemic field of study that is grounded in the discipline of nursing and informed by related fields" (Watson and Smith 2002:456). When one places Caring within an ethical science model, it automatically grounds the phenomenon as a values-laden, relational ethic that informs the ontology and the epistemology, reversing the negative mythology of epistemology put forth by Palmer. As the philosopher Levinas (1969) reminds us, ethics becomes the first principle and thus informs our ontology and epistemology rather than the other way around. The fact that nursing deals with phenomena of human caring, relationships, health-illness, living, dying, pain, suffering, and all the vicissitudes of human existence forces nursing education and practice to acknowledge and further develop an expanded view of science.

To ground nursing within the principles of *Caritas* in a Caring Science model, we can say that biomedical science and its objectivist epistemology and separatist ontology are invited once again to take account of "the face" of the other, the uniqueness of others. A purely objectivist epistemology is blind to the face wherein individuals are subsumed into units of comparison in which the difference of the other is marginalized because it cannot be expressed in such a language, in the *epistemic purpose/objectivist epistemology* of such a language. In other words, the irreducible difference of the other, the face, is indeed reduced to and becomes invisible in the universality of the care, which echoes Palmer (2004). Following Levinas, an inevitable violence has been done, an injustice that is difficult to reconcile. In a Caring Science model, "the case" must be cognizant of "the face," and it is "the face" in the first and last instances of a caring ethic and professional practice. Likewise, the Caring Science ontology is not one of distance and separation but one of relationship, purpose, connection, and meaning-making with the other, the personal face behind the impersonal patient-other.

This view has obvious implications and indeed challenges for nursing as a caring profession and for an educational ethos that would seek to promote this ethic and worldview. It is in this respect that the Levinasian notion of the dialectic of intimacy and separation of other is "reconciled in the Unity of the system" (Levinas 1969:150).

As Levinas put it, "[T]he welcoming of 'the face' is peaceable from the first, for it answers to the unquenchable Desire for Infinity" (1969:150). At the same time, this separate other yet "presence of 'the face' [of other] includes all the possibilities of the transcendent relationship" (1969:155). This understanding helps us make new connections between Levinas's notion of "the face" and the transcendence of transpersonal caring—a welcoming of "the face" in a caring moment, connecting with the infinite field of universal Love in the moment (Watson 1985).

With this understanding, Levinas's views take us, in education and practice, beyond the purely scientific model back to the face and the inexhaustible dimensions of our shared humanity in *Caritas Nursing,* in teaching and learning in a new way. In practical terms, it invites a constant questioning and revising of educational programs, curricula, health care policies, institutional regulations (where one size fits all), assessment procedures, and use of "evidence." It leads us beyond nursing as a subset of medical sciences while still being part of them and indeed merging with them but also informing them with a deep moral foundation for science.

This leads to the issue of what kind of curriculum can sustain such a *Caritas* aspiration and inspiration.

In a world like ours . . . individual authenticity lies in what we can find that is worth living for. And the only thing worth living for is Love. . . . The love that can make us breathe again, love a great and beautiful cause, a wonderful vision. A great love for one another, or for the future.

BEN OKRI (1997:57)

A Caring Science/*Caritas* orientation to nursing education intersects with arts and humanities and related fields of study, beyond the conventional clinicalized and medicalized views of human and health-healing. For Nightingale, "[N]ursing involved a sense of presence higher than the human, a 'divine intelligence that creates, sustains, and organizes the universe—and our awareness of an inner connection with this higher reality'" (Macrae 1995, quoted in Watson 2005:63). Her views, along with Levinas and his philosophy, invite us to "face our humanity" and our connectedness with the greater, infinite dimensions of our life and work.

In embarking upon a model of Caring Science/*Caritas* for nursing education, we create open space to allow evolved human consciousness to enter our phenomena, opening to notions of *Caritas/Love and Infinity* of the human spirit (Levinas 1969; Watson 2005; Watson and Smith 2002).

In Levinas's view, the life source is Infinite Cosmic Love as the Originary Primordial Love, the basis of existence of all living things. For Levinas, "[T]his is not meant to be anti-intellectual" (1969:109) but rather to lead to the very development of intellect.

Thus, this line of thinking makes a case for an underlying metaphysical-philosophical-ethical foundation for nursing rather than reverting to classical assumptions of science and knowledge and the technologies of teaching and learning. This view also reflects an evolutionary perspective for the nursing profession and the nature of knowledge itself.

> Nature and history are not just about the survival of the fittest, but
> also about the survival of the wisest . . . and the most aware.
>
> BEN OKRI (1997:133)

This evolution honors the reality that having information is not necessarily knowledge, that knowledge by itself does not necessarily lead to understanding, and that understanding is not the same as wisdom or wisdom seeking (Watson 20005). This view invites us to an awakening of an evolving human consciousness of *Caritas*, honoring the differences between stages of knowing while moving toward wisdom and integration of the whole.

As we reconsider nursing within a broader ethic-ontology-epistemology-cosmology, we realize that our approaches to our learning and teaching and practices have been too small and limiting to allow for respect of the deeper aspects of our work. In other words, our jobs have been too small with respect to the deep nature of the work nurses do (Watson 2005). Thus, our educational and epistemological and ethical models have to rise to the twenty-first-century occasion as a moral invitation and responsibility to create new or at least different educational and pedagogical options for science and society alike.

PROFESSIONAL NURSING EDUCATION FOR TOMORROW
A Values-Based Framework for *Caritas Nursing*:
Philosophy and Science of Caring

> As we examine our truth of Belonging-Being-Knowing and Doing
> Caring-Healing work in the world, how can we any longer bear to
> sustain and perpetuate an empty, hollow model?
>
> WATSON (2005:67)

Caring Science–Caritas Counterpoints to the Dominant Mythology. Without uncovering the myths and models for change, Palmer pointed out that we will always allow ourselves to be the changed and never the changers. This perpetuates the illusion that we can teach and reach into any domain we wish, manipulate and control it at a distance, without ever allowing that domain to speak back to us in a compelling way.

Caring Science and *Caritas Consciousness* help reframe and reclaim our values and the deep longings that can be integrated into our science, epistemology, and education and teaching-learning practices. Reflecting back on Parker Palmer's thesis about the mythology of epistemology—the acknowledgment that epistemology is ethic—he posed counterpoints to the dominant myth that fit within the Caring Science / *Caritas* framework (Palmer 2004:8–9):

- Every way of knowing becomes a way of living; thus, epistemology becomes ethic.

- Epistemology as ethic is a set of values to live by, a way to conduct our lives.

- Behind this reframed ethic is a way of knowing that is Personal.

- Truth is personal, radically personal, not abstract, at arm's length, propositional, "out there."

- Knowledge and knowing are communal; movement toward truth is a communal movement, with conflicts, dialogue, debates, dialectical movement toward consensus; truth emerges between and among us.

- Knowledge and knowing are about mutuality and reciprocity; truth seeks us rather than us seeking truth (Einstein talked about "listening to the universe speak"; there is a reciprocal dance between the knower and the knowing).

- Knowledge and knowing are transformational in that knowledge and seeking knowing, being challenged to seek truth, change one's life, causing one to live life more fully and deeply.

- Knowing, teaching, learning, and caring transform my knowing, teaching, and learning if they are guided by the images and norms posed here.

As Palmer reminds us (2004:9), the reason intellectual revolutions occur is related to the fact that we are increasingly uncovering these issues as myths—only as myths and not as actual truths of the world of nature, of science, of knowledge, of knowing, teaching, learning. These myths disempower people by making them think they are attempts to manipulate and control them, to make a claim on their lives. The current intellectual revolutions in caring-healing-health knowledge and practices and Caring Science frameworks are catching up with us. We have to face the fact that whether we like it or not, whether we agree with it or not, we are personally involved in transforming live encounters with the world through our scholarship, our knowledge, and our forms of teaching and learning—hence a new curriculum model.

Relationship-Centered Caring as an Educational Caring Science Core

An ethic, ontology, and epistemology of *Caritas*, of caring-healing, love, and expanded views of health and nursing, are related to a worldview of the personal, the interpersonal, the intersubjective, the intimate, the infinite, the communal, a process of mutuality-reciprocity and transformation. All of this becomes the basis for changing and being changed by the nature of our Being-Becoming in the world. This emerging Caring Science epistemology-as-ethic is grounded in relationship-centered caring and an expanded consciousness of the power of teaching.

The transformation-learning literature (Bache 2001) has noted that words we use in teaching-learning, theories, and interpretations carry much power to influence others. Words not supported by the energy of personal experiences have much less power than words grounded in personal experience that possess the energy of love and caring. In this model, higher-energy thoughts such as love and caring bring higher-frequency energy into the learning space, even if the space is nonlocal (Bache 2001). While the power of the teacher is critical to create the consciousness of a community of scholars and co-learners, the more important power is the power of the group, the community, the learning circle. Thus, the individual and collective involvement in one's own learning influences the strength and energetic stream that underpin the content (Bache 2001; Watson 2002a).

CONCLUSION

In this chapter I have extended the notion of the Carative Factor/ *Caritas Process* of teaching-learning. I have focused on the need for transformative thinking to underpin professional nursing education and a caring/*Caritas* curriculum. I have posited that the foundation of nursing as a profession lies in human relationships and caring (*Caritas*), that these qualities should form the epicenter of nursing curricula, and that all other knowledge and skills necessary for nursing practice should take account of these qualities.

Following Palmer's proposal of a "mythic epistemology," it was noted that although the objectivist biomedical sciences and evidence are obviously necessary and beneficial features of good patient care, they are not only insufficient but can, if universally dominant, distort the image of healing *Caritas* relationships in which nursing is embedded. To help make philosophical sense of this, I turned to aspects of the work of Emmanuel Levinas and his highlighting the importance of *Caritas*—love or caring for the other that goes beyond the self. For the other, Levinas uses the image of "the face." In using that image, Levinas is inviting us to consider the permanent tension that arises between a universal other and the irreducible difference of the other, upon whom a universally applied approach can inflict harm. Levinas's point is that the difference of each "face" cannot be reduced to or captured in universal aspirations and approaches. In the maxim "one size fits all—such as 'the case,'" the face is not seen; it becomes invisible. It is that which can be objectively ascertained that counts, not the face itself, not *this* individual human being. In the end, *Caritas Consciousness* seeks to give the person back to self, to see the face that stands before us. In this respect a Caring Science grounded in *Caritas* seeks to bring the objectivist epistemology of "the case" or the remote, detached impersonal policy or the economic worldview back into the face.

This "bringing back" is not simply a contrived synthesis; it is a metaphysics in the sense that it seeks not to transcend the vagaries and constraints of actual education and practice. It is intended to establish a foundation from which the knowledge and skills of nursing can emerge from an educational ethos deduced from the primary values of *Caritas,* from a broader Caring Science context. A Caring Science is not a unitary thing, a singular and rule-bound belief system. It engages with the diversity of the sciences and humanities and with notions of personal growth, of transformative learning by which the terms in which people think and the words they speak can actually be changed in educative situations. This takes time and trouble, or, put more forcefully, it takes a personal commitment by educators to enliven the importance of human relationships and caring as the epicenter of what nursing actually means, as its first and necessary condition.

Such an approach applies also to our students so we can see their "faces" and our "faces" can be seen by them, and we are seen to practice what we teach. This is not easy. As noted, it takes a certain aspiration and inspiration, what is ultimately a metaphysical worldview that recognizes and accommodates the tensions that will be met along the way. For Levinas, a relation between the self and the other is always asymmetrical, one "in which each side of the relation is 'other' for the other side" (quoted in Joldersma 200:181; also see Chinnery 2001). This applies to both educator-student and student-educator relations. If we treat our relations with others merely as roles, there is a danger of collapsing back into a universally objectivist mode of thinking in which the educative relation has no face—this student, this lecturer, this patient, this nurse, this doctor, but no face, no other, no unique individual.

There is a profound irony here in that a full lecture theater is often referred to as "a sea of faces" when in fact it is often the opposite, a crowd of no faces in which "one lecture fits all," just as one justice fits all or one science fits all. This highlights the importance of authentic dialogue in small-group interactions as part of a caring/*Caritas* curriculum. But it also alerts us to the danger that even in small-group teaching, the focus may be on what is to be learned and not on a deeper exchange within the face-to-face, human-to-human encounter—an exchange that is required if a more transformative learning experience is to occur. Joldersma described it this way:

> Thus, what is central in my role as a teacher to the student as other is responsibility. I have an obligation more primary than any freedom. In fact it might not be too strong to argue that my singularity as a teacher comes into existence through my exposure to the student as other. Here the otherness of the student can be characterized as uniqueness, something that transcends my categorization. The uniqueness of the student is actually a call to me for assuming responsibility to that person. I am responsible to her [sic] precisely because s/he is irreplaceable in the pedagogical relationship,

regardless of how many others there are. At this moment, to that person, I am responsible. That student, whose face I see, is irreplaceable, calling me to respond. This obligation is mine, personally. (Joldersma 2001:186–187)

A challenge indeed, but also an aspiration/inspiration that both calls into question and seeks a way through the political, economic, and techno-rational infrastructures that increasingly weigh us down in the name of quality that searches for universal standards, whether in learning and teaching, research, administration, or curriculum planning and implementation. These same infrastructures also weigh on students in terms of assessments, progress reports, and research or project proposals. There is a very real sense in which such infrastructures are a necessary feature of the education that takes place in universities and other educational institutions so they can operate as "going concerns," driven as much by competition and survival as by cooperation. However, such systems and those who operate passively within them, just as in objectivist science or universal systems of justice, can become blind to "the face" in the search for the universal good.

Caritas educators of nurses and health care professionals thus face a double challenge in establishing, promoting, and maintaining human-to-human dialogue and caring relationships as the epicenter of the curriculum and of teaching. As noted, this applies not only to an ethos of the practice of health care but also to an ethos that permeates the education of health care practitioners, hence the double challenge of a philosophy and science of caring for education.

The Relationship-Centered Caring (RCC) Model for Health Professions (Tressolini and Pew Fetzer Task Force 1994) serves as a guide for a Caritas curriculum that considers teaching-learning within a new paradigm. It addresses RCC educational ideals for all health professions. This curriculum model outlines some of the context and content consistent with a Caritas curriculum and an epistemology-as-ethic approach to teaching-learning.

Since the publication of my 1979 work, the philosophy and science of caring has continued to evolve through my various publications, global interactions, professional activities, relationships, and diverse speaking engagements. In the past half decade or so, caring theory as a guide for transforming clinical practice has evolved into advanced clinical models of caring scholarship and professional practices. This work is transforming self and systems as nurses reengage and more fully actualize nursing within a caring-healing, Caring Science context. Thus, in small and grand ways, nursing is being transformed from the inside out through these changes. Some of these changes have been initiated by Magnet hospital projects, but others are grass-roots changes made by staff nurses, nursing managers, visionary nursing administrators, visionary deans of nursing, and nursing faculty leaders.

As a result of this shift, the philosophy and theory of human caring is being implemented in a variety of diverse and creative scholarly ways around the United States and in other parts of the world, in both education and practice. These methods include the development of caring curricula and caring-healing professional practice models. Some of these activities are highlighted as exemplars that point to new possibilities for systems and individuals within a Caring Science context.

Examples include projects whereby ethical, theory-guided professional caring models seek to make explicit the caring relationship, knowledge, values, philosophy, therapeutics, and pedagogies that guide advanced nursing. Further, in most instances these projects are deepening the spiritual dimension of nursing.

A select group of international nurses suggested in May 2007 that an Order of Caritas Nurses be established in the future. Such a group would make explicit nurses' intentional commitment and devotion to human caring as the highest gift to humanity, their vow to practice within this consciousness and informed evolution by offering their healing gifts and deep level of humanity, opening self and other (and even systems) to the infinite field of universal Love in their work and their world.

Perhaps such an evolution will occur as we enter a new era in human history. In an earlier period of nursing history, everyone knew what a "Nightingale Nurse" was—the general consciousness and preparation of a Nightingale Nurse was different and distinguishable from those of an ordinary nurse. Likewise, in the future it is possible that a *Caritas Nurse* will have distinguishing characteristics, whereby the public will want to have *Caritas Nurses* caring for them.

ADDENDA

I. Examples of Inter/National Sites Advancing Caring Science
II. Charter: International Caritas Consortium (ICC)
III. Draft of Working Document on "Caritas Literacy" ICC Project
IV. International Caring Data Research ICC Projects
V. The Watson Caring Science Institute

*Examples of Inter/National Sites Advancing Caring Science**

While I am not and cannot be aware of all the systems using my work in a variety of ways, I am offering sites and locations that have contacted me or that I have been in contact with over the past several years. These locations and sites have indicated they are using my work in Caring Theory as a guide for advancing professional nursing in education, practice, and/or research.

These *representative* inter/national project sites are identified as places where, to my knowledge, this work is being advanced. More specific information and contact resources for the nature and direction of the

---

* Please note that these sites represent systems and activities related to the Caring Theory. I cannot be assured that they are current; in addition, the sites are likely not inclusive, as I learn every day of new places using this work.

work can be found at these Web sites: www.uchcsc.edu/nursing/caring; www.caritasconsortium.org; and www.watsoncaringscience.org.

Arizona

Grand Canyon University, Phoenix
John C. Lincoln North Mountain Hospital, Phoenix
Mayo Clinic, Phoenix
Scottsdale Health, Scottsdale
University of Phoenix, multiple campuses, Phoenix

Arkansas

University of Arkansas Children's Hospital, Little Rock

Australia

Edith Cowan University, Perth
Southern Cross University, Queensland
University of Adelaide, Adelaide
The University of Notre Dame, Fremantle

Brazil

University of Federal of Ceara, Fortaleza
University of Rio, Rio de Janeiro
University of Santa Catarina, Florianopolis

California

Kaiser Vallejo Medical Center, Vallejo
Santa Barbara City College, Santa Barbara
Scripps Memorial Hospital, La Jolla
Simpson University, Redding
St. Joseph Hospital, Orange
Stanford Hospital and Clinics, Sanford
University of California, Irvine Medical Center, Orange

Canada

Baycrest Gerontology Center, Toronto
Princess Margaret Children's Hospital, Toronto
Université du Québec, Montreal, Québec
University of Montreal, Quebec

University of Victoria, British Columbia
University of Windsor, Windsor, Ontario
York University, Ontario

China: People's Republic of China (PRC);
Republic of China (ROC) (Taiwan)
Chang Gung University, Taipei, ROC
Hong Kong Polytechnic University Kowloon, Hong Kong, PRC
Taiwan University, School of Nursing College of Medicine,
Taipei, ROC
University–Shanghai, Jiao Tong University, Shanghai, PRC

Colombia
Universidad del Norte, Barranquilla
Universidad del Valle, Cali
Universidad Nacional de Colombia, Bogotá

Colorado
The Children's Hospital, Denver
Denver Veterans' Administration Hospital, Denver
McKee Medical Center, Banner Health, Loveland
Vail Valley Medical Center, Vail

Connecticut
Greenwich Hospital, Greenwich
Middlesex Hospital, Middletown

Denmark
Aalborg University Teaching Hospital, Aalborg
Arhus University, Arhus

Finland
Abo Akademi, Department of Caring Science, Vasa
Helsinki Polytechnic, Health Care Sector, Helsinki
Helsinki University Central Hospital, Helsinki

Florida

Baptist Health, Jacksonville
Florida Atlantic University, Boca Raton
Kendall Regional, Miami
Memorial Hospital West, Pembroke Pines
Memorial Regional, South Florida
Mercy Hospital, Miami
Miami Baptist, Miami
Sarasota Memorial Health Care System, Sarasota
Tampa University Community Hospital, Tampa
Winter Haven Hospital, Winter Haven

Georgia

Memorial Health University Medical Center, Savannah
Saint Joseph's Hospital, Atlanta

Germany

Bildungswerk des Verbandes, Klostering, Irsee
German Institute of Humanistic Nursing, Bavaria

Illinois

Lake Forest Hospital, Lake Forest
MacNeal Hospital, Berwyn
Resurrection Health, Chicago
St. Mary's Hospital, Decatur
Trinity Regional Health System, Rock Island

Indiana

Family Practice Residency, Theology and Psychology
Department, University of Notre Dame, South Bend
St. Mary's Medical Center, Evansville

Indonesia

University of Indonesia, Jakarta

Iowa

University of Iowa Hospital System

Italy

Universita Bicocca, Monza
Universita Cattolica of Torino, Torino
Universita Statale, Piacenza
University of Turin, Turino

Japan

Japanese Mental Care Association, Tokyo
Japanese Red Cross College of Nursing, Tokyo
Japanese Red Cross University, Hiroshima College of Nursing,
    Hiroshima
Mie University, Mie

Kentucky

Baptist East Hospital, Louisville
Bellarmine College, Louisville
Central Baptist Health, Lexington

Korea

Catholic University School of Nursing, Seoul

Lebanon

St. Joseph's University, Beirut

Louisiana

Baton Rouge General Hospital, Baton Rouge
Our Lady of the Lake Hospital, Baton Rouge

Maine

Franklin Memorial Hospital, Farmington

Maryland

Holy Cross Hospital, Silver Spring
Union Memorial Hospital Medstar Health, Baltimore

Massachusetts

Hebrew Life, Boston

Mexico

University of Chihuahua College of Nursing, Chihuahua
University of Sonora, Hermosillo

Minnesota

The Mayo Clinic, Rochester

Missouri

Missouri Western State University, St. Joseph

Nebraska

Nebraska Methodist College of Nursing, Omaha

New Hampshire

The Cheshire Medical Center, Keene

New Jersey

AtlantiCare Regional Medical Center
CentraState Medical Center, Freehold
Monmouth Medical Center, Long Branch
Newark Beth Israel Medical Center, Newark
St. Joseph Medical Center and St. Joseph's Hospital, Paterson

New Mexico

Northern Navajo Medical Center, Shiprock

New York

Elmhurst Hospital, New York Center Health and Hospitals,
    Flushing
Highland Hospital, Rochester
Queens Hospital Center Health and Hospitals, Jamaica
Roswell Park Cancer Institute, Buffalo
St. Luke's Hospital, Newburgh
University of Rochester Strong Memorial Hospital, Rochester
Upstate Hospital, Syracuse

New Zealand

Otago Polytechnic University, Duneden

Victoria University of Wellington, Wellington

North Carolina

Moses H. Cone Memorial Hospital, Greensboro

University of North Carolina Hospitals, Chapel Hill

North Dakota

Lake Forest Hospital, Grand Forks

University of North Dakota, College of Nursing, Grand Forks

Norway

Haukeland University Hospital, Bergen

Ohio

The Ohio State University Health System, Columbus

Oklahoma

Oklahoma State University, Oklahoma City

Peru

Catholic University, Santo Toribio de Mogrovejo, Chiclayo

Philippines

Brokenshire College, Santos City

College of Nursing of Dadiangas University, Santos City

Portugal

Azores University of Terceira: Escola Superor Enferemagem do
    Heroismo, Terceira Azores (Portugal Island)

Escola Superior de Enfermagem, Cluny Maderia

University of Lisbon, Lisbon

South Carolina

Bon Secours St. Francis, Charleston

Francis Marion University, Florence

Greenville Health System, Greenville

University of South Carolina, Upstate, Spartanburg

Spain

College of Nursing (Col'legi d'Infermeria de Barcelona),
Barcelona
Santa Madrona College of Nursing, Barcelona
University of Barcelona Nursing, Barcelona
University of Tarragona, Tarragona

Sweden

Göteborg University, Göteborg
Orebro University, Department of Caring Sciences, Orebro
School of Health Sciences, Hogskolan, Boras

Switzerland

Webster University, Ballaigues

Tennessee

Mountain States Health Alliance, Johnson City

Texas

Seton Hospitals, Austin

Thailand

The Innovation Education Development Center,
Borommarajonnai College of Nursing, Pra-Buddhabat
Praboromrajchanok Institute for Health Workforce
Development, Ministry of Public Health, Saraburi Province
Prince of Songkla University, Songkla Province
Saint Louis Nursing College, Bangkok

United Kingdom

City University, London
University of Bedfordshire, Luton

Utah

Weber State University, Ogden

Venezuela

Carabobo University, Valencia

Virginia

Inova Health System, Fairfax and Falls Church

St. Mary's Hospital, Bon Secours Healthcare System, Richmond

Washington, DC

The Catholic University

West Indies

University of West Indies School of Nursing, Kingston, Jamaica

West Virginia

City Hospital, Martinsburg

Mountain State University, Beckley

Wisconsin

Alverno College, Milwaukee

Vitebo University, La Crosse

Wyoming

Wyoming Medical Center, Casper

Charter: International Caritas Consortium

As a result of recent national and international developments in the use of Caring Science Theory and Philosophy of Human Caring as a guide to transformative work in nursing scholarship, education, and practice, a gathering of invited professionals is emerging. These are committed professionals who are authentically being-doing and advancing the work in the world and who wish to convene to deepen the *Caritas Model*, share their activities, and learn from each other.

The group has named itself the International Caritas Consortium. Different institutions using this model host gatherings of these likeminded professionals upon invitation from me. All are from institutions in which the new caring-healing models are being implemented, along with selected others who are advancing Caring Science scholarship and practices. Anyone interested in participating can contact me at jean.watson@uchsc.edu. Additional information is on the Caritas

Consortium Web site, www.caritasconsortium.org, and my Web site: www.uchsc.edu/nursing/caring.

Sponsors of the International Caritas Consortium to date are:

- University of Colorado Health Sciences Center, Denver, Colorado
- Miami Baptist, Miami, Florida
- Resurrection Health System, Chicago, Illinois
- Inova Health, Fairfax, Virginia
- Central Baptist Health, Lexington, Kentucky
- Scripps Health, La Jolla, California
- Bon Secours Health, Richmond, Virginia
- Scottsdale Health, Scottsdale, Arizona

Projected sponsors include:

- Jacksonville Baptist Health, Jacksonville, Florida
- Memorial Bon Secours Health, Charleston, South Carolina
- Casper Medical Center, Casper, Wyoming

INTERNATIONAL CARITAS CONSORTIUM (ICC) CHARTER

Purpose

The main purposes of this emerging International Caritas Consortium are:

1. To explore diverse ways to bring the caring theory to life in academic and clinical practice settings by supporting and learning from each other; and

2. To share knowledge and experiences so that we might help guide self and others in the journey to live the caring philosophy and theory in our personal/professional life.

The consortium gatherings will:

- Provide an intimate forum to renew, restore, and deepen each person's, and each system's, commitment and authentic practices of human caring in their personal/professional life and work;

- Learn from each other through shared work of original scholarship, diverse forms of caring inquiry, and model caring-healing practices;

- Mentor self and others in using the Theory of Human Caring to transform education and clinical practices;

- Develop and disseminate Caring Science models of clinical scholarship and professional excellence in the various settings in the world.

Membership

The participants of the Caritas Consortium are invited representatives of clinical and educational systems and/or selected individuals who are advancing the education, professional practice, and research of Caring Science/Human Caring Theory through their respective role and activities in the USA and various locations in the world.

Structure-Coordination: Core Caritas Coordinating Council (CCCC)

The Core Caritas Coordinating Council serves as a subgroup of the membership and functions as a coordinating and communicating body with the members. The core members will include:

- Dr. Jean Watson, founder of the original Theory of Human Caring, who serves as Chair/Honorary Chair;

- Selected representatives from original leadership member representatives from organizations/systems developing and advancing the model of caring theory and practices throughout their institution.

The council shall consist of six or fewer members, who will provide continuity and stability; coordinate the agendas; and provide leadership for emerging projects of the ICC.

Meetings

The ICC members and new invitees shall meet in the spring and fall of each year, per the sponsorship of member(s) who request to host the gathering. The host institution and its representatives shall serve as the primary organizing/agenda-setting body for the gathering in their institution, along with assistance from previous hosts, the Core Caritas Coordinating Council, and Dr. Watson.

Responsibilities/Activities for Gatherings

- Provide a safe forum to explore, create, renew self and system through reflective time out.

- Share ideas, inspire each other, and learn together.

- Participate in use of Appreciative Inquiry whereby each member is facilitative of each other's work, each learning from others.

- Create opportunities for original scholarship and new models of caring-based clinical and educational practices.

- Generate and share multi-site projects in caring theory scholarship.

- Network for educational and professional models of advancing caring-healing practices and transformative models of nursing.

- Share unique experiences for authentic self-growth within the Caring Science context.

- Educate, implement, and disseminate exemplary experiences and findings to broader professional audiences through scholarly publications, research, and formal presentations.

- Envision new possibilities for transforming nursing and health care.

Draft of Working Document on "Caritas Literacy" ICC Project*

CARITAS LITERACY

Caritas "Literacy" is used instead of the more technical term "competencies" to acknowledge that caring and caritas consciousness encompasses unique attributes. These human and humane attributes include an intentional, cultivated, and learned approach of the whole person to have "fluency" and learned skills of emotional and heart-centered intelligence, knowledge, and skillful ways of Being Human; to cultivate a consciousness evolution that opens up the higher level energetic, infinite spiritual field of one's humanity.

---

* Reprinted with permission of working subgroup from International Caritas Consortium (June 2007). (Subgroup of International Caritas Consortium: Gene Rigotti, Joanne Duffy, Jim D'Alfonso, Teri Woodward, Jean Watson.) Modified by Jean Watson, January 30, 2008.

"Others" refers to all people one encounters—patients, families, visitors, co-workers, volunteers, everyone; every race, color, creed, nationality, and lifestyle.

CARITAS CONSCIOUSNESS

Practicing loving kindness and equanimity within the context of caring consciousness. *My respect for this patient (other) allowed me to be available to him/her.*

- Opens to connectedness with self, others, environment, and universe.
- Models self-care and caring for others.
- Validates uniqueness of self and others.
- Acknowledges acts of kindness (i.e., seeds etc.).
- Honors own and others' gifts and talents.
- Recognizes vulnerabilities in self and others.
- Treats self and others with loving kindness.
- Listens respectfully and with genuine concern to others.
- Accepts self and others as they are.
- Demonstrates respect for self and others.
- Listens to others.
- Treats others with kindness.
- Pays attention to others.
- Respects others.
- Honors the human dignity of self and others.

Being authentically present and enabling and sustaining the deep belief system of self and one being cared for. *By listening, I was able to honor this patient's (other's) belief system and enable him/her to feel his/her own sense of faith/hope.*

- Creates opportunities for silence/reflection/pause.
- Promotes intentionality and human connections with others
- Views life as a mystery to be explored rather than a problem to be solved.

- Able to release control to higher power.
- Interacts with caring arts and sciences to promote healing and wholeness.
- Incorporates others' values, beliefs, and what is meaningful and important to them into the care plan.
- Utilizes appropriate eye contact and touch.
- Calls others by their preferred names.
- Helps others to believe in themselves.
- Supports others' beliefs.
- Supports others' sense of hope.
- Encourages others in their ability to go on with life.

Cultivating one's own spiritual practices and transpersonal self, going beyond ego-self (working from a more full consciousness of heart-centeredness—opening to all chakras, including fourth chakra and above). *By being more responsive to the patient's (other's) needs and feelings, I was able to create a more trusting-helping-caring relationship.*

- Practices self-reflection (journaling, prayer, meditation, artistic expression), demonstrates willingness to explore one's feelings, beliefs, and values for self-growth.
- Practices discernment in evaluating circumstances and situations vs. being judgmental.
- Develops meaningful rituals for practicing gratitude, forgiveness, surrender, and compassion.
- Transforms "tasks" into caring-healing interactions.
- Accepts self and others on a basic spiritual level as unique and beautiful beings worthy of our respect and caring.
- Is able to bless and forgive self and others.
- Demonstrates genuine interest in others.
- Values the intrinsic goodness of one's self and others as human beings.

Developing and sustaining helping-trusting authentic caring relationships. *I develop helping-trusting caring relationships with patients (others), families, and members of the health care team.*

- Enters into the experience to explore the possibilities in the moment and in the relationship.
- Holds others with unconditional love and regard.
- Seeks to work from the other's subjective frame of reference.
- Holds a sacred space of healing for others in their time of need.
- Practices nonjudgmental attitudes.
- Responds to others with congruence to others' lived experience.
- Practices authentic presence:
  - Brings full, honest, genuine self to relationship.
  - Demonstrates sensitivity and openness to others.
  - Engages in I-Thou relationships vs. I-It relationships.
- Demonstrates awareness of own and others' style of communications (verbal and nonverbal).
- Seeks clarification as needed.
- Promotes direct, constructive communication:
  - Engages in communication that promotes healthy living; does not engage in gossip.
  - Engages in effective, loving communication; does not engage in rumors.
  - Engages in proactive problem solving; does not engage in chronic/excessive complaining.
  - Engages in activities that maximize independence and individual freedom; does not engage in inappropriate dependence.
  - Engages in activities that promote safe, ethical, mature, healthy growth experiences; does not engage in unethical, illegal, safety-risk, or seductive behavior.
- Allows others to choose the best time to talk about their concern(s).

Being present to, and supportive of, the expression of positive and negative feelings as a connection with deeper spirit of self and one-being-cared-for. *I co-create caring relationships in caring environments to promote spiritual growth.*

- Creates/holds sacred space (safe place for unfolding and emerging).

- Acknowledges healing as an inner journey.
- Allows for uncertainty and the unknown.
- Encourages narrative / storytelling as a way to express understanding.
- Allows for story to emerge, change, and grow.
- Encourages full expression of sensations, feelings, thoughts, ideas, emotions, beliefs, and values to explore understanding and meaning.
- Encourages reflection of feelings and experiences.
- Offers blessings, prayer, and spiritual expression as appropriate.
- Helps others see some good aspects of their situation.
- Actively listens and lets energy flow through one's self without becoming consumed by other's feelings.
- Accepts and helps others deal with their negative feelings.

Creatively using self and all ways of knowing as part of the caring processes; engaging in artistry of caring-healing practices. *I exercise other-centered problem solving and scholarship in caring for this patient (other).*

- Integrates aesthetic, ethical, empirical, personal, and metaphysical ways of knowing with creative, imaginative, and critical thinking for full expression of caring arts and sciences.
- Acknowledges and integrates an awareness that the presence of oneself is to be included as an effective element of the plan of care for others.
- Uses self to create healing environments via:
  - Intentional Touch
  - Voice
  - Authentic presence
  - Movement
  - Art–artistic expression
  - Journaling
  - Play-laughter-gaiety
  - Spontaneity
  - Music-sound
  - Preparation
  - Breathing

- Relaxation-imagery-visualization
- Thoughts-consciousness-intentionality
- Appropriate eye contact
- Smiling, positive gestures
- Active listening
- Heart awareness (what we hold in our hearts is energetically being communicated)
- Nature, light, sound/noise protection
- Others

- Encourages others to ask questions.

- Helps others explore alternative ways, to find new meaning in their situations/life journeys in dealing with their health/self-healing approaches.

Engaging in genuine teaching-learning experiences that attend to unity of being and meaning, attempting to stay within another's frame of reference. *The co-created caring relationship promotes knowledge, growth, empowerment and healing processes and possibilities for patients (others) and for self.*

- Actively listens with one's whole being to others' relaying of their life experiences.

- Speaks calmly, quietly, and respectfully to others, giving them full attention in that moment.

- Seeks first to learn from others, understand their worldview; then shares, coaches, and provides information, tools, and options to meet others' needs (works from others' frame of reference).

- Participates in collegial/collaborative co-creation.

- Accepts others as they are and where they are with their understanding, knowledge, readiness to learn.

- Helps others understand how they are thinking about their illness/health.

- Asks others what they know about their illness/health.

- Helps others formulate and give voice to questions and concerns to ask health care professionals.

Creating healing environment at all levels (physical as well as non-physical, subtle environment of energy and consciousness) whereby wholeness, beauty, comfort, dignity, and peace are potentiated. *By promoting the caring relationship I created space for this patient (other) to generate his/her own wholeness and healing.*

- Creates space for human connections to naturally occur.
- Participates in caring-healing consciousness.
- Creates caring intentions.
- Creates a healing environment attending to:
  - Nurse as environment
  - Other as unique person
  - Light
  - Art
  - Water
  - Noise
  - Cleanliness
  - Privacy
  - Nutrition
  - Beauty
  - Safety
  - Hand washing
  - Comfort measures
  - Others' time frames
  - Others' routines and rituals
- Is available to others.
- Pays attention to others when they are talking.
- Anticipates others' needs.

Assisting with basic needs, with an intentional caring consciousness; administering "human care essentials," which potentiate alignment of mind-body-spirit, wholeness and unity of being in all aspects of care. *I was able to help meet the needs this patient (other) identified for him/herself.*

- Views others as integrated whole.
- Respects others' unique individual needs.
- Makes others as comfortable as possible.

- Helps others feel less worried.
- Is responsive to others' family, significant others, loved ones.
- Makes sure others get the sustenance they need.
- Respects others' need for privacy.
- Respects others' perceptions of the world and their unique needs.
- Involves family / significant others.
- Treats other's body carefully as mystery of participating in life force of another.
- Helps others with special needs for relaxation, restoration, and sleep.
- Talks openly to family.

Opening and attending to spiritual-mysterious and existential dimensions of one's own life-death; soul care for self and the one-being-cared-for. *I allow for miracles to take place with self and others.*

- Allows for the unknown to unfold.
- Participates in paradox of life.
- Surrenders control and anticipates miracles.
- Nurtures / supports hope.
- Shares and participates in human caring moments as appropriate.
- Acknowledges one's own and others' inner feelings.
- Knows what is important to self and others.
- Shows respect for those things that have meaning to others.
- Believes that fundamental love and good abounds in all situations where life exists.

International Caring Data Research ICC Projects

INTERNATIONAL CARING COMPARATIVE DATABASE
Duffy—CAT

The International Caring Comparative Database (ICCD) is a dynamic repository that began as a scholarly endeavor associated with the International Caritas Consortium (ICC). This group of health professionals is connected through the use of caring theory in a clinical-practice-research relationship.

The ICCD is an open and flexible database managed by Joanne Duffy PhD, RN, FAAN (Principal Investigator) of The Catholic University of America in Washington, DC. The database collects and evaluates patients' perceptions of nurse caring behaviors from health care institutions throughout the world. Using the CAT-version IV (Duffy, Hoskins & Seifert, 2007)[1] and some patient descriptors (e.g. age, gender, educational level), participating institutions receive unit-level comparative data reports to use for benchmarking, seeking out best practices, quality improvement, and research.

The ICCD stores the nursing-sensitive *process* indicator, nurse caring behaviors. Other process indicators, such as nurse manager caring behaviors and nurse educator caring behaviors may be added. These indicators of caring provide participating institutions with timely information about the experience of care (from the patient, staff nurse, and student points of view). Regularly assessing caring processes allows clinicians, educators, and administrators to monitor improvements in nursing practice, to link caring processes with nursing-sensitive outcomes measures, to study ways that structural indicators such as staffing patterns or nurse credentials affect caring processes and to examine trends over time.

The ICCD is the only comparative database of caring behaviors performed by nurses. It has grown from an "idea" to a reality because health care institutions' that use caring theory as basis for new professional practice models, and as a foundation for advancing nursing practice, are actively seeking ways to research, connect and improve their services.

To participate in the ICCD, health care institutions can contact Dr. Joanne Duffy at 202-319-6466 or duffy@cua.edu and agree to join for one year, participate in a one-hour training program (on-site), collect data quarterly through a random selection process, and receive and disseminate quarterly reports for practice improvement.

Institutions will receive quarterly reports of their data compared to other institutions and trended over time. No unique identifiers will be used so anonymity and confidentiality is assured. Opportunities to provide feedback and assistance with publication/presentation ideas will be provided.

The Watson Caring Science Institute,(WCSI) a new non-profit foundation, created to serve and extend the scholarly activities of the ICC, can serve as an additional funnel for communicating, expanding, and disseminating this global caring database.

THE CARING INTERNATIONAL RESEARCH COLLABORATIVE

Nelson—CPS

The Caring International Research Collaborative was initiated to connect multiple specialty research groups for the purpose of sharing and exploring how their respective areas of research connect with one another. The goal of the collaborative is to create a Structural Equation Model (SEM), which is a model that explains how variables within the health care environment interact to impact patient outcomes, including perception of caring. One of the instruments used as part of this activity is the Caring Factor Survey, which was designed to assess caring within the context of Watson's theory of caring and recent work in Caritas nursing (www.uchsc.edu/nursing/caring).

Recent research in caring from this collaborative has identified that nurses who are reported to be most caring by the patients they care for provide the most consistent care, are nurses with the most professional nursing experience, are most affected emotionally by the patient, do not work overtime, are from every age category, and are most frustrated with the work environment, especially workload (Persky et al. 2008). The 2007 international database, which includes over 500 patients from Italy, the Philippines, and the United States, revealed that among the caring factors, nurses were consistently rated highest in conveying loving kindness to their patient and lowest in tending to the spiritual needs of patients. This measurement will assist with theory testing and refinement of the caring process.

Continued validation of measurement of caring is planned by relating the patients' reports of feeling cared for to blood components that are present when they feel stressed (cortisol), love (DHEA), and physically resilient (IgA). Understanding how the patients' report of feeling cared for relates to their physical state goes beyond validating measurement of caring to articulate the relationship this feeling has to healing. This challenge will require measurement of other variables that likely influence healing, including the environmental aspects from which nurses, physicians, and other care providers work.

Factors that are currently being examined in relationship to caring include workload, primary nursing, management, competence, knowledge management, HeartMath, caring, HIV/AIDS, Healthcare

Environment Survey (HES), staffing, floating, nurse report, overtime, position control, rapid response team, sitters, management, competence, education, lean management, patient safety and relationship-based care. Countries involved as of January 2008 are the Bahamas, Belgium, Brazil, Cameroon, England, Ireland, Italy, the Philippines, Serbia, Switzerland, Tanzania, and the United States.

A hierarchical approach is used among the participants to understand how these variables and others persist in multiple settings across the globe, and how they operate within each country and each participating facility. This group may find that caring is a moderating factor of other clinical and organizational results.

The group's rapid growth and effective dialogue over the last two years, growing from 4 to over 130 members, has been attributed to interest in the phenomenon of caring as well as caring for each other. Members serve each other using their unique talents, whether administrator, researcher, educator, clinician, or consultant. It is the hope the rigorous scientific methods with open sharing will support the evolvement of caring as a vital element of healing for not only the patient but also the care providers and health care environments alike at a global, national and facility level.

The Caring Factor Survey Scale can be downloaded from Watson's Web site: www.uchsc.edu/nursing/caring. To understand more about this group and the research on caring and the Caring Factor Survey instrument and other health care measures, contact John Nelson.

John W. Nelson
President, Healthcare Environment
888 West County Road D., Suite 300
New Brighton, MN 55112 USA
Office Phone: 651-633-4505
Mobile Phone: 651-343-2068
Skype Phone: 651-314-4505
Fax: 651-633-6519
jn@hcenvironment.com
www.hcenvironment.com

NOTE

1. The Caring Assessment Tool (CAT—version IV) determines the degree of nurse caring as perceived by patients. It is a theoretically-based instrument taken from Watson's *Theory of Human Caring* (1979; 1985). The instrument has been revised twice, first to allow for use in multiple settings and secondly to evaluate reliability and establish construct validity (Duffy et al, 2007). The questions are directed at how nurses perform specific activities within the healthcare situation. Responses indicate how frequently an activity occurs. The CAT consists of 36 items and is designed to be completed by the recipient of care (the patient).

The Watson Caring Science Institute

TRANSFORMING HEALTH CARE
ONE NURSE / ONE PRACTITIONER AT A TIME

The Watson Caring Science Institute (WCSI) is an international non-profit foundation created to advance the philosophies, theories, and practices of human caring, originated by Distinguished Professor Jean Watson, who holds the Murchinson-Scoville Endowed Chair in Caring Science at the University of Colorado Denver and Health Sciences Center. The Theory and Science of Human Caring seeks to restore the profound nature of caring-healing and bring the ethic and ethos of Love back into health care. Through an extended network of professional, clinical, and academic colleagues, the WCSI will translate the model of caring-healing/*Caritas* into more systematic programs and services that will continue to transform health care one nurse / one practitioner / one educator / one system at a time.

The WCSI is dedicated to helping the current health care system retain its most precious resource—competent, caring professional nurses—while preparing a new generation of health professionals within a broader model of Caring Science. The WCSI will help to ensure caring and healing for the public, reduce nurse turnover, and decrease costs to the system.

The WCSI intends to:

1. Create a professional network of Caring Science / *Caritas* Practitioners, who bring profound caring-healing and Love back into health care.

2. Provide a vehicle for the continuing development, implementation, and integration of Caring Science / *Caritas* clinical-educational programs, modeled by the developer, Distinguished Professor Jean Watson, PhD, RN, FAAN, and through a network of professional, clinical, and academic colleagues.

3. Support and archive the continued development of Dr. Watson's lifetime of esteemed work in Caring Science as the foundation for sustaining caring-healing for practitioners, patients, and the public, thus facilitating transformation of nursing and the health care system.

4. Honor "first" donor individuals and organizations at WCSI Charter Sponsor Members with a privilege package forthcoming.

We are the light —

Jean Watson

POSTSCRIPT: PRESCRIPT

You do not know this yet—but
You are already
Being and Becoming a *Caritas Nurse* as you engage in this work

You are entering into what nursing has always been
But has yet to fully realize.

Carry forth your vision of caring and healing;
Continue to follow your heart, head, and actions
Into untrod and untried places and spaces

Challenge and more fully actualize
Your personal/professional gifts and talents

Respond to your inner call for compassionate caring and healing
        for self and others
Access your Source for practices that sustain you and your humanity

May you be blessed with guidance as you
Choose each step

I am honored to be a sojourner with you on
This path we create and walk together
Continually unfolding in the universe of possibilities

The end and the beginning

Ackerknecht, E. H. (1968). *A Short History of Medicine.* New York: Ronald, 1968.

Aiken, L. H., H. K. Smith, and E. T. Lake. (1994). Lower Mortality Among a Set of Hospitals Known for Good Nursing Care. *Med. Care* 32:771–787.

Arrien, A. (2005). *The Second Half of Life.* Boulder, CO: Sounds True.

Astin, J. (1991). *Remembrance* (compact disc). Santa Cruz, CA: Golden Dawn Productions.

Bache, C. (2001). *Transformative Learning.* Sausalito, CA: Noetic Sciences Institute.

Bent, K., et al. (2005). Being and Creating Caring Change in a Healthcare System. *International Journal of Human Caring* 9(3):20–25.

Bjerg, S. (2002). Jakob Knudsen. Totality Through Life Experience. In R. Birkelund, ed., *Existence and Philosophy of Life.* Copenhagen: Gyldendal.

Blegen, M. A., and T. A. Vaughn. (1998). A Multisite Research of Nurse Staffing and Patient Occurrences. *Nursing Econ.* 16(4):196–203.

Boyce, J. (2007). Nurses Making Caring Work: A Closet Drama. Unpublished PhD dissertation. Victoria University, British Columbia, Canada.

Boykin, A., and S. Schoenhofer. (2001). *Nursing as Caring: A Model for Transforming Practice.* New York: National League for Nursing.

Buber, M. (1958). *I and Thou,* 2nd ed. New York: Scribner's.

Chinnery, A. (2001). Asymmetry and the Pedagogical I-Thou. In *Philosophy of Education Yearbook.* Champaign: University of Illinois at Urbana-Champaign.

Chodron, P. (2005). *No Time to Lose.* Boston: Shambhala.

Dossey, B. M., L. Keegan, and C. Guzzetta. (2005). *Holistic Nursing: A Handbook for Practice,* 4th ed. Boston: Jones & Bartlett.

Dossey, L. (1991). *Meaning and Medicine.* New York: Bantam.

———. (1993). *Healing Words, the Power of Prayer and the Practice of Medicine.* San Francisco: Harper.

Duffy, J. (1992). The Impact of Nurse Caring on Patient Outcomes. In D. Gaut, ed., *The Presence of Caring in Nursing.* New York: National League for Nursing.

———. (2002). Caring Assessment Tools. In J. Watson, ed., *Instruments for Assessing and Measuring Caring in Nursing and Health Sciences.* New York: Springer Publishing.

———. (2003). The Quality-Caring Model. *Advances in Nursing Science* 26(1): 77–88.

Duffy, J., L. Hoskins, and R. F. Seifert. (2007). Dimensions of Caring: Psychometric Properties of the Caring Assessment Tool. *Advances in Nursing Science* 39(3):1–12.

Emerson, R. W. (1982). *Ralph Waldo Emerson: Selected Essays.* New York: Penguin American Library.

Erikson, E. H. (1963). *Childhood and Society.* New York: Norton.

Eriksson, K. (1999). *The Trojan Horse.* Vasa, Finland: Abo Akademi, Insitutionen for Vardvetenskap.

Foucault, M. (1975). *The Birth of the Clinic: An Archaeology of Medical Perception.* Trans. A. M. Sheridan Smith. New York: Random/Vintage Books.

Frankl, V. E. (1963). *Man's Search for Meaning.* New York: Washington Square Press.

Greene, M. (1991). Texts and Margins. *Harvard Educational Review* 61(1):25–39.

Halldorsdottir, S. (1991). Five Basic Modes of Being with Another. In D. A. Gaut and M. Leininger, eds., *Caring: The Compassionate Healer.* New York: National League for Nursing.

Harman, W. W. (1990–1991). Reconciling Science and Metaphysics. *Noetic Science Review* 40:5–10.

———. (1991). *A Re-examination of the Metaphysical Foundation of Modern Science.* Sausalito, CA: Institute of Noetic Sciences.

———. (1998). What Are Noetic Sciences? *Noetic Science Review* 47:32–33.

Hanh, Thich Nhat. (2003). *Creating True Peace.* New York: Free Press.

Heidegger, M. (1962). *Being and Time.* New York: Harper and Row.

———. (1971). The Nature of Language. In M. Heidegger, ed., *On the Way to Language.* New York: Harper & Row.

Herman, K. (1993). Reassessing Predictors of Therapist Competence. *J. Counseling Dev.* 72(5):29–32.

Hesse, H. (1951). *Siddhartha.* Trans. Hilda Rosner. New York: New Directions.

Horvath, A. O., and B. D. Symonds. (1991). Relation Between Working Alliance and Outcome in Psychotherapy: A Meta-Analysis. *Journal of Counseling Psychology* 38(2):139–149.

Housden, R. (2005). *How Rembrandt Reveals Your Beautiful, Imperfect Self.* New York: Harmony Books.

Jarrin, O. (2006). An Integral Philosophy and Definition of Nursing: Implications for a Unifying Theory of Nursing. Unpublished manuscript, July.

Joldersma, C. W. (2001). Pedagogy of the Other: A Levinasian Approach to the Teacher-Student Relationship. In *Philosophy of Education Yearbook.* Champaign: University of Illinois at Urbana-Champaign.

Kabat-Zinn, J., and M. Kabat-Zinn. (1997). *Everyday Blessings.* New York: Hyperion.

Kandinsky, W. (1977). *Concerning the Spiritual in Art.* New York: Dover.

Kaplan, S. H., S. Greenfield, and J. E. Ware. (1989). Assessing the Effects of Physician-Patient Interactions on the Outcomes of Chronic Disease. *Medical Care* 27(Suppl. 3):S110–S127.

Kluckholn, C. M., H. A. Murray, and D. M. Schneider, eds. (1953). *Personality in Nature, Society and Culture.* New York: Knopf.

Kornfield, J. (2002). *The Art of Forgiveness, LovingKindness, and Peace.* New York: Bantam.

Kovner, C. T., and P. J. Gergen. (1998). Nurse Staffing Levels and Adverse Events Following Surgery in US Hospitals. *Image. J. Nursing Scholarship* 30:315–321.

Lafo, R. R., N. Capasso, and S. R. Roberts. (1994). Introduction. Body and Soul: Contemporary Art and Healing. In *Body and Soul: Contemporary Art and Healing.* Lincoln, NE: De Cordova Museum.

Leininger, M. M. (1981). *Caring: An Essential Human Need.* Thorofare, NJ: Charles B. Slack.

Levin, D. (1983). The Poetic Function in Phenomenological Discourse. In W. McBride and C. Schrag, eds., *Phenomenology in a Pluralistic Context.* Albany: State University of New York Press.

Levinas, E. (1969). *Totality and Infinity.* Pittsburgh, PA: Duquesne University (14th printing, 2000).

Logstrup, K. (1997). *The Ethical Demand.* Notre Dame, IN: University of Notre Dame.

Luborsky, L., P. Crits-Cristophy, and A. T. McClellan. (1986). Do Therapists Vary Much in Their Success? Findings from Four Outcome Studies. *American Journal of Orthopsychiatry* 56(4):501–512.

Macrae, J. A. (2001). *Nursing as a Spiritual Practice.* New York: Springer.

Malkin, J. (1992). *Hospital Interior Architecture: Creating Healing Environments for Special Patient Populations.* New York: Van Nostrand Reinhold.

Martin, D. J., J. P. Garske, and K. M. Davis. (2000). Relation of the Therapeutic Alliance with Outcome and Other Variables: A Meta-Analytic Review. *J. Consulting Clinical Psychol.* 68(3):438–450.

Martinsen, K. (2006). *Care and Vulnerability.* Oslo, Norway: Akribe.

Maslow, A. H. (1968). *Toward a Psychology of Being.* Princeton, NJ: Van Nostrand.

Mitchell, S. (1994). *A Book of Psalms.* New York: HarperPerennial.

Muff, J. (1988). Of Images and Ideals: A Look at Socialization and Sexism in Nursing. In A. H. Jones, ed., *Images of Nursing: Perspectives from History, Art, and Literature.* Philadelphia: University of Pennsylvania.

Myss, C. (1996). *Anatomy of the Spirit: The Seven Stages of Power and Healing.* New York: Harmony Books.

Newman, M. (1994). *Health as Expanding Consciousness.* Philadelphia: F. A. Davis.

Newman, M., A. M. Sime, and S. A. Corcoran-Perry. (1991). The Focus of the Discipline of Nursing. *Advances in Nursing Science* 13:1–14.

Nightingale, F. (1969). *Notes on Nursing: What It Is and What It Is Not.* New York: Dover.

Okri, B. (1997). *A Way of Being Free.* London: Phoenix.

Orlinsky, D. E., and K.I.L. Howard. (1985). Therapy Process and Outcome. In S. Garfield and A. Bergin, eds., *Handbook of Psychotherapy and Behavior Change.* New York: John Wiley & Sons.

Palmer, P. (1987). Community, Conflict and Ways of Knowing. *Magazine of Higher Learning* 19:20–25.

————. (2004). *The Violence of Our Knowledge: Toward a Spirituality of Higher Education.* 21st Century Learning Initiative. Kalamazoo, MI: Fetzer Institute.

Pew Fetzer Report. (1994). See Tressolini, C. P., and Pew-Fetzer Task Force.

Persky, G., Nelson, J. Watson, J., et al. (2008). "Creating a Profile of a Nurse Effective in Caring." *Nursing Administration Quarterly* 32(1): 15-20.

Plath, S. (1962). "Tulips." In *Ariel* by Sylvia Plath. Harper & Row.

Quinn, J. F. (1989). On Healing, Wholeness and the Haelan Effect. *Nursing and Health Care* 10(10):553–556.

————. (1992). Holding Sacred Space: The Nurse as Healing Environment. *Holistic Nursing Practice* 6(4):26–35.

————. (1997). Healing: A Model for an Integrative Health Care System. *Advanced Practice Nursing Quarterly* 3(1):1–7.

————. (2000). Transpersonal Human Caring and Healing. In B. Dossey, ed., *Holistic Nursing: A Handbook for Practice*, 3rd ed. Gaithersburg, MD: Aspen.

Quinn, J., M. Smith, C. Ritenbaugh, K. Swanson, and J. Watson. (2003). Research Guidelines for Assessing the Impact of the Healing Relationship in Clinical Nursing. *Alternative Therapies in Health and Medicine* 9(3) (Suppl.):A65–A79.

Roach, M. S. (2002). *Caring, the Human Mode of Being: A Blueprint for the Health Professions*, 2nd ed. Ottawa: Catholic Health Association Press.

Rogers, M. E. (1970). *A Theoretical Basis of Nursing.* Philadelphia: F. A. Davis.

————. (1994). The Science of Unitary Human Beings. *Nursing Science Quarterly* 2:33–35.

Rosenberg, S. (2006). Utilizing the Language of Jean Watson's Caring Theory Within a Computerized Clinical Documentation System. *CIN: Computers, Informatics, Nursing* 24(1):53–56.

Rotter, J. B. (1954). *Social Learning and Clinical Psychology.* Englewood Cliffs, NJ: Prentice-Hall.

Rumi, J. (2001a). *Hidden Music.* Trans. M. Mafi and A. Kolin. London: Thorsons/HarperCollins.

————. (2001b). *The Glance: Rumi's Songs of Soul Meeting.* Trans. C. Barks. New York: Penguin Compass.

Ryan, L. (2005). The Journey to Integrate Watson's Caring Theory with Clinical Practice. *International Journal of Human Caring* 9(3):26–30.

Samueli Conference on Definitions and Standards in Healing Research. (2002). San Diego, CA.

Sartre, J. P. (1956). *Being and Nothingness.* New York: Philosophical Library.

Schlitz, M., E. Taylor, and N. Lewis. (1998). Toward a *Noetic* Model of Medicine. *Noetic Science Review* 48:45–52.

Schultz, W. C. (1967). *Joy: Expanding Human Awareness.* New York: Grove.

Shattell, M. (2002). Eventually It'll Be Over: The Dialectic Between Confinement and Freedom in the Phenomenal World of the Hospitalized Patient. In S. Thomas and H. Pollio, eds., *Listening to Patients: A Phenomenological Approach to Nursing Research and Practice.* New York: Springer.

Smith, M. (1992). Caring and the Science of Unitary Human Beings. *Advances in Nursing Science* 21(4):14–28.

Solomon, R. C., and K. M. Higgins. (1997). *A Passion for Wisdom: A Brief History of Philosophy.* Oxford, UK: Oxford University.

Strupp, H. H., and S. W. Hadley. (1979). Specific vs. Nonspecific Factors in Psychotherapy: A Controlled Study of Outcome. *Archives of General Psychiatry* 35(10):1125–1136.

Swanson, K. (1999). What Is Known About Caring in Nursing Research: A Literary Meta-Analysis. In A. S. Hinshar, S. Feetham, and J. Shaver, eds., *Handbook of Clinical Nursing Research.* Thousand Oaks, CA: Sage.

Tarnas, Richard. (2006). *Cosmos and Psyche: Intimations of a New World View.* New York: Viking.

Tolle, E. (1999). *The Power of Now.* Novato, CA: New World Library.

———. (2003). *Stillness Speaks.* Novato, CA: New World Library.

Tolstoy, L. (1889). *My Religion.* London: Walter Scott.

———. (1889 [1968]). *The Wisdom of Tolstoy.* Trans. Huntington Smith. New York: Philosophical Library. An abridgement.

Tressolini, C. P., and Pew Fetzer Task Force. (1994). Health Professionals Education and Relationship-Centered Care. San Francisco: Pew Health Commission.

van den Berg, J. H. (1966). *Psychology of the Sickbed.* Pittsburgh: Duquesne University Press.

Vaughn, F. (1995). *Shadows of the Sacred: Seeing Through Spiritual Illusions.* Wheaton, IL: Quest Books.

Walker, L. O., and K. C. Avant. (2005). *Strategies for Theory Construction in Nursing,* 4th ed. Englewood Cliffs, NJ: Pearson Education/Prentice-Hall.

Watson, J. (1979). *Nursing: The Philosophy and Science of Caring.* Boston: Little, Brown. Reprinted/republished 1985. Boulder: Colorado Associated University Press.

———. (1985). *Nursing: Human Science and Human Care, a Theory of Nursing.* Norwalk: CT: Appleton-Century-Crofts. Reprinted/republished 1988.

New York: National League for Nursing. Reprinted/republished 1999. Sudbury, MA: Jones & Bartlett.

———. (1997). The Theory of Human Caring: Retrospective and Prospective. *Nursing Science Quarterly* 10(1):49–52.

———. (1999). *Postmodern Nursing and Beyond*. Edinburgh, Scotland: Churchill-Livingstone. Reprinted/republished 2005. New York: Elsevier.

———. (2002a). Intentionality and Caring-Healing Consciousness: A Practice of Transpersonal Nursing. *Journal of Holistic Nursing Practice* 16(4): 12–19.

———. (2003). Love and Caring: Ethics of Face and Hand. *Nursing Administration Quarterly* 27(3):197–202.

———. (2004a). Caring Science Web site: www.uchsc.edu/nursing/caring.

———. (2004b). Commentary: Relational Core of Nursing Practice. *Journal of Advanced Nursing* 47(3):241–250.

———. (2005). *Caring Science as Sacred Science*. Philadelphia: F. A. Davis.

———. (2006). Caring Theory as Ethical Guide to Administrative and Clinical Practices. *Nursing Adm. Quarterly* 30(1):48–55.

———. (2008a) The International Caritas Consortium Web site: www.caritasconsortium.org (under construction).

———. (2008b) The Watson Caring Science Institute Web site: www.watsoncaringscience.org (under construction)

———, ed. (2002b). *Assessing and Measuring Caring in Nursing and Health Science*. New York: Springer.

Watson, J., and M. Smith. (2002). Caring Science and the Science of Unitary Human Beings: A Transtheoretical Discourse. *Journal of Advanced Nursing* 37(5):452–461.

Weber, R. (1986). *Dialogues with Scientists and Sages: The Search for Unity*. London: Routledge & Kegan Paul.

Wilber, K. (1998). *The Essential Ken Wilber*. Boston: Shambhala.

———. (2001a). *A Theory of Everything*. Boston: Shambhala.

———. (2001b). Web site: http://wilber.shambhala.com/html/misc/haberman/index.cfm/xid,5837/yid,5049275.

Williamson, M. (2002). *Everyday Grace*. New York: Riverhead.

Yalom, I. D. (1975). *Theory and Practice of Group Psychotherapy*, 2nd ed. New York: Basic Books.

Young, S. (2006). Web site: http://shinzen.org.

THE WATSON CARING SCIENCE INSTITUTE

presents

Caritas Meditation

Featuring the Spoken Messages of Jean Watson

& the Music of Gary Malkin

1. *Caritas* Meditation
2. *Caritas* Prayer
3. The Caring Moment©
4. Music Meditation: Letting Yourself Be Loved©

Tracks 1 & 2 co-produced 2008 by Jean Watson and Gary Malkin; Watson Caring Science Institute and Wisdom of the World; music composed & arranged by Gary Malkin; assisted by Dan Alvarez Musaic Studios, Berkeley, California. www.musaic.biz; www.wisdomoftheworld.com; www.watsoncaringscience.org.

Track 3 with permission from *Care for the Journey.* www.careforthejourney.net; www.companionarts.org.

Track 4 with permission from *Graceful Passages: A Companion For Living and Dying.* www.wisdomoftheworld.com.

For more information on how to obtain other resources by Jean Watson, go to www.uchcsc.edu/nursing/caring; www.caritasconsortium.org; and www.watsoncaringscience.org.

For more information on how to obtain the musical resources of Gary Malkin, go to www.wisdomoftheworld.com.

The
Watson Caring
Science Institute

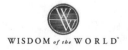

WISDOM *of the* WORLD